Mental Health Professionals in Medical Settings

A Primer

Mental Health Professionals in Medical Settings
A *Primer*

JoEllen Patterson, Ph.D.
C. J. Peek, Ph.D.
Richard L. Heinrich, M.D.
Richard J. Bischoff, Ph.D.
Joseph Scherger, M.D., M.P.H.

W. W. Norton & Company, Inc.
New York • London

For information about permission to reproduce
selections from this book, write to
Permissions, W. W. Norton & Company, Inc.,
500 Fifth Avenue, New York, NY 10110

Book design and composition by Paradigm Graphics
Manufacturing by Haddon Craftsmen

Library of Congress Cataloging-in-Publication Data

Mental health professionals in medical settings : a primer / by JoEllen
    Patterson ... [et al.].
        p.   cm.
    Includes bibliographical references and index.
    ISBN 0-393-70338-X
    1. Mental health services—United States—Handbooks, manuals, etc. 2.
    Mental health personnel—United States—Handbooks, manuals, etc. 3.
    Holistic medicine—United States—Handbooks, manuals, etc. I.
    Patterson, JoEllen

    RA790.6 .M4435 2002
    362.2'0973—dc21   00-050050

W. W. Norton & Company, Inc., 500 Fifth Avenue, New York, NY 10110
www.wwnorton.com

W. W. Norton & Company Ltd., 10 Coptic Street, London WC1A 1PU

1   2   3   4   5   6   7   8   9   0

The authors wish to thank Brenda Lee, M.A., for her amazing editing and organizational help. Without her perseverance and gentle prodding, this book would never have been written.

Contents

Introduction

The Medical-Mental Health Split in Health Care—What We Can Do About It

One of the most significant events in the history of health care has been the development of separate and parallel systems of mental and medical care. However, patients want and need integrated physical and mental health care. This book is about how mental health professionals can change their practices to bridge the gap between medical and mental health care in medical settings.

The following facts illustrate the importance of integrating mental health care into the primary care setting (Chudy & Dea, 1996; Pincus et al., 1998; Regier, Goldberg, & Taube, 1978; Regier et al., 1993; Shapiro et al., 1984; Shi, 1992; Strosahl, 1997).

- Fifty percent of mental health care is delivered solely by primary care physicians.
- Sixty-seven percent of all psychopharmacological drugs are prescribed by primary care physicians.
- Ninety percent of the 10 most common complaints in the primary care setting have no organic basis.
- Fifty to 70% of all primary care visits are primarily for psychosocial concerns.
- In recent years, approximately 7% of patients visiting their primary care provider received psychotropic medications.
- Only a small percentage of the population of patients with mental disorders or emotional distress will ever see a mental health professional.

Over the past 20 years an emerging body of research literature and clinical experience has suggested promising methods for bridging the traditional gulf between medical and mental health care (Ford, 1994). Such comprehensive and well-coordinated care that encompasses both the biomedical and psychosocial aspects of health and illness is often called integrated care.

Our own efforts in this regard have followed a course of discontent, discovery, and experimentation: discontent when fragmented systems of health care "carve up" the patient and his treatment; discovery, in finding that despite our diverse backgrounds and specialties, we shared a singular goal and could learn to speak each other's language; and experimentation, in asking new questions of ourselves and our disciplines, and trying "outside the box" solutions for more comprehensive patient care.

Indeed, we have worked in both fragmented and integrated systems of health care and have experienced the unfortunate consequences of fragmented care. As a result, we have dedicated our professional efforts to creating alternative, integrative clinical approaches where patients receive the total care that they need, especially where that care needs to bridge the biomedical and psychosocial aspects of health and illness. We represent multiple health care specialties including family medicine, psychiatry, health psychology, and marriage and family therapy. We also work in four different health care delivery settings in various areas of the United States. Our diverse backgrounds in training and work settings, coupled with a shared vision of integrated health care, have strengthened each of our efforts to achieve collaborative care for our patients.

While each of us felt that the expertise from our particular discipline made significant contributions to our patients' well-being, we began to feel uncomfortable limiting our work to the confines of our training and discipline. Instead of asking what our discipline offered our patients, we began asking, "What do our patients need?" We were aware of the burgeoning body of literature linking mental health to genetics and biology; however, we were looking beyond biological explanations of mental health problems. Instead, we wanted to understand how biological, psychological, and social influences interact to create unique situations and struggles for each patient. For example, how does the patient with a history of depression cope with receiving a diagnosis of prostate cancer? How can we best help the diabetic patient who complains about her emotionally empty marriage and eats poorly when she feels depressed? What do we have to offer a senior patient who has a history of heart disease, is newly widowed, and is barely functioning because he is so overwhelmed with grief? What do we offer the patient who is burdened and discouraged by chronic headaches but who has no diagnosable psychopathology or organic disease?

During this process we noticed a chasm between the medical health care world and the mental health care world. We tried to figure out ways to cross that chasm because we felt that this was the best way to provide optimal care for our patients. In the process, we have had to change the way we practice and *think* about our work. For example, we no longer hold allegiance to the 50-minute hour. Similar to the primary care physician, we take as long as we need but no more. We might have an hour-long visit with a family whose father is dying of lung cancer and a 20-minute visit for the mother and bed-wetting child. But regardless of the time that we spend, the patient's needs always come first, and thus guide the choices we make. In addition, we frequently extend our attention and questions to areas beyond our traditional disciplines and ask for help from our diverse colleagues. Because we are members of very different professions, we have had to make extra efforts to talk to each other and understand the language and culture of the other disciplines.

Many ideas presented in this book are based on literature documenting that most patients with mental health problems, psychological distress, or stress-linked physical symptoms initially present their concerns in a primary care setting and are never seen by a mental health clinician. In fact, because of this phenomenon the primary care setting is commonly referred to as the *de facto mental health care delivery system* (Regier et al., 1978, 1993). Primary care physicians pride themselves on treating "the whole patient," but despite their best intentions are often unable to fully understand and treat their patients' mental health concerns. This is mostly due to the fact that there is little time for the physician to address much beyond the patient's physical complaint. The result is that patients' mental health needs can be overlooked. Smoothly incorporating mental health and social factors into the care of illness or injury and into the improvement of health is often very difficult for patients and clinicians, and most of this difficulty is because of the legacy of separate and parallel systems of care (National Committee for Quality Assurance, 1998, 1999; Strosahl, 1998).

Causes of Fragmented Health Care

The mind-body split that is played out in separate and parallel systems for physical and mental health care is nothing new. The notion of body as distinct from mind and soul dates back centuries to the time of Galileo, Newton, and Descartes (Engel, 1992b). Such historical precedents laid the foundation for the dual views of health care that took root over the last hundred years. Today, physicians and mental health professionals usually practice in separate settings, focus on either body or mind, and ask different types of questions to arrive at a diagnosis and develop a treatment plan. This split also has had a major influence in the world of finance and insurance reimbursement where there are separate guidelines and fee schedules for what is covered. In many plans, reimbursement depends on meeting criteria for a specific diagnosis, and generally physical and mental diagnoses are distinct.

Organizationally and economically this has led to mental health care being "carved out" from the overall medical benefit in many health insurance plans. Although initially this was as a strategy to provide more benefits to the insured, over time it has developed as a method for controlling rising mental health costs and restricting primary care physicians' ability to provide comprehensive mental health treatment when they are competent to do so. Many factors, including historical, philosophical, economic, and business influences, as well as health care professionals' training philosophies, and patients' attitude caused this dichotomy to develop.

Business and economics encourage fragmentation of care. Health care organizations set standards for the number of patients a physician sees daily and appointments are made at set intervals. Economic incentives exist for time- and cost-efficient practices. If a patient has a specific biomedical problem, the physician prescribes the appropriate treatment and moves on to the next appointment with the satisfaction of having met the previous patient's needs. Because of set time constraints, it is easier and more expedient for the physician to stay focused on one or two clearly defined biomedical problems. In a system where patients are allotted 10–15 minutes for a visit, multiple vague patient problems can be overlooked (Plocher & Kongstvedt, 1998).

The traditional practice and training strategy in both medical and mental health care emphasizes the mind-body split. In its most polarized and stereotypical characterization, medical professionals are trained to address the physical health of patients. Although the patient's emotional and psychological health may exacerbate physical symptoms, they can be ignored, missed, overlooked, or not dealt with directly. In fact, physicians sometimes view physical health as distinct and separate from the emotional and psychological issues impacting a person's functioning. Likewise, mental health professionals sometimes address the emotional and psychological health of their patients without regard to physical condition. Many mental health practitioners view mental health disorders as their exclusive domain.

Training programs also contribute to the mind-body split. Until recently, mental health training programs did not require students to take courses in health psychology, neurobiology, physiology, and pharmacology. Although medical schools and residency programs have long required behavioral science courses and training, they are typically not given the status of other courses that are considered more practical in nature. From the time physicians begin their medical education, they are taught to value the skill and knowledge of the specialist. This mind-body split also continues in medical practice as the administrative support and time commitment needed to support collaborative relationships are lacking.

Patients themselves are not immune to dividing concerns over health and illness into separate physical and mental domains, often to their detriment. A significant reason for this is that patients bring with them a history of receiving health care. Every interaction that the patient has had with physicians and psychotherapists informs this history and their perception of the health care delivery system. News and popular media have a strong influence on a patient's perceptions as well. Because a person's perception is shaped by news stories about patients being misdiagnosed or mistreated by the health care system, patients may be more demanding and less trustful of health care professionals after exposure to these stories. As a result, a patient's history of experience and perceptions of others' experiences influence the roles and treatment within the physician-patient relationship. In addition patients are often reluctant or unable to identify feelings such as sadness, worry, or loneliness. These patients may be more comfortable offering physical complaints and will ignore the accompanying emotions, thus perpetuating the status quo of fragmented care.

Common Dissatisfaction with Fragmented Care

The current disconnected systems of health care delivery often force providers and patients to choose between medical and behavioral health care, even when the clinical picture calls for a blend of the two. Because treatment of human health and illness does not neatly break down into traditional "either-or" delivery structures, dissatisfaction is often felt by all those involved. Appendix A presents examples of complaints we have heard over the years while doing clinical work and conducting consultations with patients, clinicians, clinics, and care systems (Peek & Heinrich, 2000).

Identifying patients with *DSM-IV-TR* (American Psychiatric Association [APA], 2000) diagnoses and referring them to outside mental health professionals only addresses part of the problem. These models leave the separate and parallel delivery structure intact by attempting to root out mental illness and substance abuse for separate behavioral health treatment. This organizational approach contrasts with what research is teaching us about the intricate relationship between physical and mental health, and if the delivery of health care continues to be separated, the benefits of this knowledge will not be fully realized.

In the past, when we were working in the current fragmented organizational system of health care delivery, we were simultaneously reading the burgeoning clinical literature demonstrating that people are whole and need holistic health care. While the financial and operational health care systems kept care fragmented, the clinical research suggested that this separation did not fit with patients' needs or with our professional aspirations.

Interaction between Physical and Mental Health

Although ancient cultures have recognized the complex interaction between physical and mental health, Western researchers are only now beginning to study and acknowledge this important interaction. For instance, research has shown how a "fighting spirit" serves as a protective factor against the recurrence of breast cancer, and a satisfying marriage protects against repeat myocardial infarction (Spiegel, 1999; Williams & Chesney, 1993). We want to briefly share some key examples of current mind-body research that has influenced our work.

A Connection between Mental and Physical Illness

Patients who are hospitalized for myocardial infarction and who suffer from major depression have an increase in mortality at six months (Carney et al., 1988). In fact, the identification of major depression as an independent risk factor was found to be "at least equivalent to that of left ventricular dysfunction and a history of previous MI [myocardial infarction]." (Frasure-Smith, Lesperance, & Talajic, 1993). Psychological distress also adversely affects prognosis in coronary patients, increasing their susceptibility to recurrence and rehospitalization (Allison et al., 1995; Gullette et al., 1997). Another example of the behavioral-physical relationship is that individuals reporting high levels of anxiety or depressive symptoms are at elevated risk for developing hypertension (Dimsdale, 1997; Glassman & Shapiro, 1998; Jonas, Franks, & Ingram, 1997; Robinson, Starr, & Price, 1984).

A Connection between Social Network and Immune System

Diverse social networks such as friends, family, work associates, and community members protect patients against upper respiratory tract illnesses such as the common cold. Social ties also increase life span, influence regulation of the immune system, and may play a role in the ability of the human body to resist infection (Cohen, Doyle, Skoner, Rabin, & Gwaltney, 1997).

A Connection between Therapy and Brain Functioning

While we do not yet understand the pathways or underlying mechanisms between psychosocial experiences and physical illness, a relationship linking these two clearly exists. As an example, behavior therapy can cause physical changes in brain activity. Specifically, behavioral treatments given to patients with obsessive compulsive disorder produced beneficial changes in the glucose metabolic rate (Baxter et al., 1992). Although future research can delineate the pathways between the psychosocial and the physical, health care practitioners do not need to wait for a complete explanation to begin incorporating these important findings into their practice and to provide holistic care for their patients.

Although health care professionals have known about the mind-body connections for a long time, health care is still not set up to treat the whole patient. In spite of the limits imposed by our health care settings, we still try to think about holistic patient care. The biopsychosocial model has been a critical tool in helping us do this.

The Biopsychosocial Model

A psychotherapist colleague of ours who works with physicians contrasts his training with theirs by saying he was taught to work with "bodyless minds" while they were taught to work with "mindless bodies." We smiled when we heard that description because it described our training. Another example of this mind-body training dichotomy often arises when we talk about family history in our clinics. The therapists in the group may be thinking about genograms, family legacies, and family-of-origin issues. The physicians may be thinking about the BRCA2 markers, hemochromatosis, trisomy 21, dopaminergic mechanisms, and A1 alleles. No wonder we have trouble understanding each other!

George Engel, a physician at the University of Rochester, has addressed this conceptual and language dichotomy. In a classic article initially published in *Science*, he raised questions about the adequacy of the biomedical model (Engel, 1977). Engel argued that the biomedical model is too limited to understand complex human phenomena and suggested that a new medical model be created—the biopsychosocial model (Engel, 1977, 1992a). In this new model there is no separation of organic and inorganic phenomena. All parts—biological, psychological, and social—work together to create a whole person and all parts influence each other, creating new interactions. For a summary of the ideas that have been most helpful to us, and an expanded definition of the biopsychosocial model, see Appendix B.

Applying the Biopsychosocial Model in the Real World of Economic and Operational Health Care Limitations

While the clinical world embraces a biopsychosocial model, the operational and financial world may be more reticent. Concerns arise about skyrocketing costs if patients with "problems of living" are reimbursed for counseling and treatment in the medical setting. Some payors require a *DSM-IV-TR* diagnosis before they are willing to pay for treatment. Other payors offer services for crisis intervention only. Suicide intervention could be paid for, but prevention of domestic violence or child abuse may not if these strict guidelines are followed. Other payors chose not to enter the debate about what should be paid for and simply set a limit on the number of sessions they will cover each year, regardless of the problem.

Although the therapist working in a medical setting does not have to know the solutions to these complex issues, he or she at least needs to be aware of the issues and the fact that there are a variety of views on how a biopsychosocial model can be implemented. Perspectives on these views also vary according to the perspective and training of each professional. For example, one clinic in San Diego was interested in doing primary care screening for mental health disorders using PRIME MD (Spitzer et al., 1994), a rapid, self-report, assessment measure that screens for the most common mental disorders in a primary care setting. Enthusiastic clinicians, hopeful of identifying previously untreated patients with mental health problems, became more cautious when they realized payors concerns: If all primary care patients were screened for mental health issues, would the cost of mental health services increase? Do all patients really need treatment, especially for their mental health concerns? Thus, while the biopsychosocial model makes excellent clinical sense, implementing it remains complex. The following section describes what has been tried so far.

Three Approaches to Behavioral Health Care

When we think about integrated health care, three approaches come to mind, each demonstrating different levels of integration:

- mental health (i.e., behavioral health) care as a specialty,
- behavioral health care integrated in primary care, or
- behavioral health care integrated in specialty care.

Behavioral Health Care As a Specialty

As a generalization, specialty behavioral health is oriented around mental health and substance abuse illnesses and problems, care is delivered in separate behavioral health clinics, and care plans are more or less focused on behavioral health disorders rather than general health care. While most health plans or insurance permits direct patient self-referral to behavioral health care, referral is the main pathway primary care physicians follow to get mental health or substance abuse assessment or therapy for their patients.

The specialty behavioral health care practitioner typically focuses on *DSM-IV-TR* diagnoses and medical necessity for treatment. In essence, the ticket for treatment is symptom severity and poor daily functioning. From this perspective, integration might involve screening for psychiatric disorders and providing referrals for behavioral health treatments. Collaboration might mean coordinating separate and parallel medical and behavioral health care plans where the behavioral health portion consists of hospitalization or medication for mental illnesses. Collaboration may also be two different professionals (i.e., a primary care physician and a mental health clinician) communicating about their shared patients and the specific problem they are each independently treating. Group or individual therapies for serious mental health or substance abuse conditions might be offered or mental health clinicians may take over patients' care from the primary care provider when mental health or substance abuse problems become severe or unusual.

Improved consultation and coordination between medical providers and mental health/substance specialists no doubt represent a big improvement over completely disconnected systems. Placing mental health providers in primary care settings is one example of improved coordination. These adjustments to the traditional specialty referral model for behavioral health care do not get to the heart of what is needed for primary care patients and physicians.

One difficulty that goes with using specialty behavioral health care (even when "attached" to a primary care site) to handle all the problems that surface in primary care is a higher threshold for patient eligibility for reimbursable behavioral health care. That is, the patient usually must have a diagnosable behavioral health disorder (i.e., a *DSM-IV-TR* diagnosis). It is common for patients to take their symptoms to a primary care physician without regard to their medical or psychological origins. As a consequence, approximately 70% of office visits to primary care physicians do not lead to a diagnosable medical illness (Strosahl, 1997). If the patient has a chronic headache or stress-linked symptoms without a diagnosable mental condition, it may be difficult for the behavioral health professional to find a reimbursable behavioral health care code, particularly if the patient is adamant that he or she has no behavioral health problems. Many subclinical states of distress, or DSM-IV-TR "V" code conditions (e.g., marital problems, family stress, job dissatisfaction) are not covered by insurance, even though they play a large part in many difficult and costly cases in primary care (Simon, Von Korff, & Barlow, 1995; Von Korff, Ormel, Katon, & Lin, 1992). In addition to being associated with high utilization of medical services, these stressors can alter physiology and lead to significant pathology (Dunman, Heninger, & Nestler, 1997; Holmes & Rahe, 1968). For example, they can lead to depression and anxiety and precipitate the course of major mood disorders (Goodwin & Jamison, 1990).

While the DSM-IV-TR code for "psychological factors affecting physical condition" can be applied broadly to these situations, the basic (and totally unnecessary) strain here is the need to legitimize behavioral health care on the basis of a separate behavioral health care benefit. A more sensible approach would be a comprehensive health care benefit that allows flexible use of various kinds of providers on the extended medical team.

From a patient service perspective, a specialty behavioral health care model requires the patient to be able and willing to articulate a mental health or substance problem (or at least follow their physician's recommendation) in order to see a mental health or chemical health professional for help. Unfortunately, many patients fail to recognize mental health symptoms and will not see a therapist for help. However, if they do reach a therapist, complaining of aches and pains or denying behavioral health problems is often a quick route back to the physician. As a result, providing a behavioral or mental explanation to a patient who cannot see it yet can be a disservice to the patient.

From a patient access perspective, if all primary care patients with a behavioral health problem were referred to specialty behavioral health care, there would not be enough psychiatrists or behavioral health clinicians to handle the load (Katzelnick, 1997). Since primary care is the de facto mental health care delivery system (Regier et al., 1978, 1993), it is unfair to patients (as well as providers) to expect the traditional specialty behavioral health care model, all by itself, to serve the behavioral health needs of a population. Specialty treatment (such as hospital, day treatment, and other therapies) for mental health and substance abuse disorders is essential but cannot be expected to effectively cope with the volume and range of psychosocially related presentations in primary care.

From a teamwork perspective, a specialty mental health model, if left to do it all, tends to reinforce mutual stereotypes and misunderstandings between primary care and behavioral health care providers, since they usually relate at a distance and work from quite different philosophies and cultures (McDaniel, Campbell, & Seaburn, 1995). With little opportunity to routinely discuss and resolve problems that do arise, misunderstandings may linger and mutual stereotypes flourish. Colocating specialty behavioral health care and primary care may improve this somewhat, but building up good teamwork, mutual trust, and rapid recovery from problems requires people to interact more routinely and more personally than usually takes place through referrals, phone calls, or even chats on the way to the parking lot.

Behavioral Health Care Integrated in Primary Care

Integrated behavioral health providers help with behavioral, emotional, or behavioral health–related factors that emerge as important in the care of primary care patients. Common areas in which integrated behavioral health providers are frequently involved are chronic illnesses, headaches, and other pain complaints; somatization or multiple vague complaints; industrial injury or worker's compensation; and comorbid mental illnesses that complicate medical treatment and adherence.

Behavioral health professionals come to the primary care clinic as long-missing members of the primary care team, and share the same broad population-based or public health mission of primary care professionals, rather than being focused on a particular disease. The work crosses the majority of medical conditions and is not characterized only by treatment for diagnosable mental disorders. Integrated behavioral health clinicians typically work out of the medical examination rooms and schedule appointments with the same receptionists and scheduling system as the physicians. They also use the same waiting room as the primary care physicians and write in the patient's medical chart in a way that respects all state and federal regulations on confidentiality.

Over a period of years, integrated behavioral health care professionals often have an important effect on primary care culture, particularly in creating change toward greater acceptance and openness regarding difficult clinician-patient relationships. In addition, behavioral health care clinicians effectively demonstrate how to form care teams and plans that make clinic practice more satisfying and ultimately lead to better outcomes (for case examples, see Lucas & Peek, 1997).

Our experience with medical and behavioral health collaboration and integration of care within medical clinics has led to the creation of flexible and long-term working relationships that employ gradations of integration depending on the needs of the specific patient, couple, or family. Overall, such collaborative relationships have been well received by our medical colleagues and patients (Fisher & Ransom, 1997). Although primary care and behavioral health professionals will have to await further research documenting effective interventions, the emerging literature suggests there is ground for collaboration, experimentation, and application of behavioral health skills and approaches adapted to the primary care setting (Mauksch et al., 2000; McDaniel et al., 1990).

Studies showing reduced morbidity and mortality in patients with heart disease or cancer who were treated with behavioral health interventions have captured the attention of the public and scientific communities (Fawzy et al., 1993; Linden, Stossel, & Maurice, 1996). Patients with heart attacks and untreated depression were 3.5 times more likely to die from another heart attack within six months after a heart attack compared to patients without depression (Frasure-Smith et al., 1993). Fawzy and colleagues (1993) found that patients with malignant melanoma who attended a six-week coping skills group had enhanced survival six years later. Spiegel, Bloom, and Kraemer (1989) also found enhanced survival for patients with advanced breast cancer who attended a support group, compared to a control group. Behavioral health professionals in primary care settings can be called upon to help manage the care of patients with a variety of medical disorders including diabetes, rheumatoid arthritis, cancer, heart disease, and hypertension.

In addition to the value of behavioral health interventions to health outcomes, an important relationship exists between behavioral health interventions and stewardship of resources. The literature on medical cost-offset is beginning to describe how some patients with psychosocial problems can overutilize health care services such as lab tests or emergency room visits (Simon et al., 1995; Unutzer et al., 1997).

Simon, Von Korff, and Barlow (1995) found large cost differences in the treatment of primary care patients with anxiety and depressive disorders, even when controlling for medical comorbidity. Essentially, the study showed that the treatments for patients with depression and anxiety were more expensive than for patients without these disorders. Cummings (1997), in the Hawaii Medicaid project, demonstrated that focused treatment rather than traditional psychotherapy can effectively manage patients referred from primary care, resulting in significant cost effects.

Behavioral Health Care Integrated in Specialty Care

The general principles and approach outlined for behavioral health integrated in primary care applies to integration with specialty care as well, but there are some important differences in emphasis, knowledge, and skills required from behavioral health professionals. Specialty care is focused sharply and intensely on a set of conditions, diseases, or organ systems for which specialty physicians and nurses develop deep knowledge and skills. Behavioral health clinicians who enter specialty settings develop correspondingly great knowledge and skills in these areas in addition to the general skills they bring to patient care of all kinds. For example, a behavioral health clinician who joins an oncology clinic will learn about the relevant issues related to cancer, both from a medical and a psychological perspective. Without developing a working understanding of what oncology physicians and nurses face, do, and make decisions about, the behavioral health clinician will not really become integrated. In the same way, behavioral health clinicians entering endocrinology clinics will learn about diabetes, and therapists entering neurology clinics would benefit from knowing about headaches and common diseases of the nervous system. Behavioral health professionals do not need to know everything about those diseases and treatments, but they need to be oriented to the key realities of the diseases, medical care, and language spoken in specialty clinics.

Challenges Facing the Integrated Behavioral Health Clinician

A behavioral health professional starting work in a primary or specialty care setting is likely to be among the first generation of mental health professionals to do so. They will most likely enter clinics or systems that contribute to some degree or another to the dissatisfactions described earlier. They might be part of a system where ambiguity remains about how behavioral health professionals are integrated into the clinic and care of its patients. Therefore, sensitivity to care system problems and issues, as well as patient problems, is especially important.

Having the ability to identify problems, empathize with medical colleagues, and develop solutions to improve patient and local care systems is essential.

Therapists are more effective when they understand what the patient and family face, what kinds of behavioral health factors or goals are associated with complications or with improved outcomes, and which care plans and techniques are most appropriate for the patient's condition and personal situation. Psychoeducational groups, couples therapy, or specific behavioral medicine techniques such as such as hypnosis, biofeedback, and relaxation training may become important tools in the therapist's "black bag."

We recognize that the primary care physician has the overall perspective and will act as the treatment team leader. We view the role of the mental health clinician as enhancing the physician-patient relationship. This means that the mental health clinician generally will remain in the background as a care team member, not as a separate and independent alternative to the primary care physician. This is important considering that many patients have significant behavioral health issues factored into their overall health concerns but are not aware of them at the outset. In fact, patients themselves may not recognize mental health factors in their medical complaints or recognize that their somatic symptoms represent emotional distress (Barsky, 1988). It is common for a patient to hold his or her entire suffering in a medical frame of reference, even when a purely medical approach has little more to offer. These patients are unlikely to seek psychotherapy on their own and are often reluctant to start off talking about personal issues.

Integrated behavioral health providers refrain from thinking that such a patient is "not a good therapy candidate," nor do they complain that "all the patient could think about was headache and fatigue." Instead, the clinicians realize that the situation calls for something besides traditional psychotherapy or psychological assessment. The situation calls for the therapists to help a patient distill a personal agenda out of a whole pot of physical suffering and anger at life or medical people while allowing the patient to retain the medical frame of reference for the suffering. This does not necessarily look or sound like psychological assessment or therapy to the patient or to the therapists. Typically, behavioral health care clinicians who have developed this part of their professional repertoire have expanded their profession beyond the traditional techniques of mental health and substance abuse therapy into a broader view of their profession.

Medical patients are not the only "customers" for integrated behavioral health. Consultation to physicians and nurses (rather than having the therapists take over the care) is very common. The goals of such consultations are to help these care providers to broaden their repertoire, to increase the effectiveness of their interventions, and to help them manage their reactions to difficult patients (Roter et al., 1995). It is not uncommon for integrated behavioral health clinicians to help medical clinic physicians and staff recognize and constructively deal with personal "buttons" pushed by particularly challenging patients in the clinic (Lucas & Peek, 1997). Behavioral health professionals also consult with primary care clinicians to prevent patients being treated for chronic pain, anxiety, or industrial injury from falling into "disability ruts."

In addition to consultation, the behavioral health clinician participates in the ongoing care of patients with chronic medical illnesses such as diabetes, asthma, and cancer when depression, anxiety, coping skills, or psychosocial factors complicate medical management, patient morale, or family coping (Miranda, Hohmann, Attkisson, & Larson, 1994). When the behavioral health care professional does handle ongoing care, it is in the context of the overall medical care plan carried out by the medical team as managed by the physician, rather than as a part of an independent behavioral health care plan. A few primary care patients have both significant medical illnesses as well as serious behavioral health diagnoses such as depression or personality disorder. While some patients might not engage well in specialty behavioral health care clinics, they can be treated by the primary care team over a period of years, with the integrated behavioral health clinician as a major figure on that care team.

Integrated behavioral health clinicians help make accurate, timely, and successful referrals to specialty behavioral health care when patients present with specific needs, or as they begin to recognize specialty behavioral health care agendas within their physical suffering (e.g., incest survivors with chronic pain). It is important to work with somatically preoccupied patients in the medical clinic until they are able to see how their personal situations affect their health or begin to accept behavioral health factors as part of the explanation for their symptoms. Only if and when such patients can articulate a need for the kind of therapy provided through specialty behavioral health care will they be referred to a specialist. This process of distilling a behavioral health care agenda out of a pot of physical suffering could be called "pre-therapy therapy," and is typically done by integrated behavioral health professionals. Specialty mental health referrals succeed only when both the patient and the clinician can articulate the purpose of the referral. In capitated care systems, the cost of integrated behavioral health tends to be thought of as part of medical costs, rather than only as behavioral health care costs. There is far more emphasis on deploying the behavioral health care professionals to exert leverage on overall health status and costs than with finding a way to generate billable behavioral health care codes or to reduce utilization of behavioral health services alone. Financial models for integrated behavioral health are probably simplest in a capitated environment, but creative ways to achieve the integrated clinical goal can be found in fee-for-service systems as well.

The Audience and Outline of this Book

While we hope that physicians will find this book useful, it is primarily written for mental health professionals from any discipline who are looking to provide more comprehensive and improved integrated care for their patients. The book will be especially relevant to mental health professionals who are working in the physical health field such as the physician's office or in a hospital setting and are interested in expanding their skills in the medical setting. We have also written this book for new mental health professionals who may be uniquely receptive to learning new ways of practicing their profession.

This book is a primer for the mental health professional working in a medical setting. In Part I we discuss health care settings. To provide a basic understanding of the differences between traditional medical and mental health care systems, we describe the specific cultures of primary care, specialty care, and mental health care (Chapters 1 and 2). In Chapter 3 we discuss ways to balance the clinical, operational, and financial perspectives of health care.

In Part II we provide information on how to build collaborative medical care. In Chapter 4, a five-stage model for the process of developing integrated care is introduced. We present the importance of expanding therapists' roles when working in the medical setting and argue that therapists should expand their thinking beyond clinical considerations (Chapter 5). In Chapters 6 through 8, we focus on specific suggestions for mental health care providers who work as part of a collaborative team in medical settings. This includes how to work within the organizational framework of the medical system (Chapter 6), models for working with common problems seen in primary care (Chapter 7), and ways to promote preventative care (Chapter 8). We conclude the book (Chapter 9) by highlighting some of the opportunities that exist for therapists to be part of an important social shift in how health care is provided.

In this book many terms for "mental health professional" are used, and are often used more or less interchangeably. To help reduce the confusion that results from the multiplicity of terms, Appendix C provides a description of these terms.

While we hope to provide readers with an understanding of the problems resulting from the separation of medical and mental health care, we also acknowledge the many challenges that remain to achieve an alternative system of care. Our goal is to share our experiences, knowledge, and vision on how to overcome these challenges so that all health care professionals have the opportunity to embrace a collaborative, multidisciplinary approach. We aim to enrich readers' appreciation of integrative health care as a viable and necessary alternative to traditional fragmented care, for the purpose of providing effective, quality care that all patients need and deserve.

Part I
ABOUT HEALTH CARE SETTINGS

Chapter 1

The Culture and Context of Primary and Specialty Health Care

The front line of health care, where patients with undifferentiated symptoms present to health care professionals, is the domain of primary care. In public health terms, *primary care* refers to the entry points into the health care system, primarily in office settings but also in homes, nursing homes, hospital clinics, and emergency rooms. *Secondary care* refers to the work of specialists and the care given in community hospitals. *Tertiary care* is provided by subspecialists in specialized hospitals or academic health centers. In this chapter we discuss the culture and context of primary and specialty health care.

Primary Care

Development of Primary Care

Historically, primary care has been provided by professionals trained to address the whole person in the context of the patient's family and community. The general practitioner is the classic primary care provider, with a tradition dating back to 500 B.C. with Hippocrates in Greece. As modern medicine has become increasingly specialized during the last half of the 20th century, primary care has seen the emergence of its own specialties.

An example of a primary care specialty is family practice. Although family practice continues the general practice tradition of addressing the health care needs of all members of a family and community, it is distinguished from general practice by the requirement of three additional years of residency training. Because this training is designed to provide the education necessary to do the job in a modern context, it includes a strong emphasis on the behavioral sciences to address psychosocial problems affecting health. Two additional types of primary care specialties that emerged during the 20th century are general internal medicine for adults and general pediatrics for children. Similar to family practitioners, these community-based primary care practitioners undergo three years of residency training after medical school.

In most of the world, primary care is still provided by general practitioners or family physicians. However, in the United States, family physicians and residual general practitioners deliver only half of primary care treatment. In fact, about half of adults and children in the United States receive their primary care from general internists and pediatricians. General obstetricians/gynecologists provide much of the primary care to women of childbearing age, even though their training is mostly surgical and limited to the reproductive organ system. White, Williams, and Greenberg, in a classic article titled "The Ecology of Medical Care" (1961), used an epidemiological analysis to show that most health problems are addressed appropriately in a primary care setting. The rapid specialization of American physicians in the 1960s and beyond raised a concern that there would not be adequate physicians to provide primary care, and the specialty of family practice was born (White, 1967).

Other health professionals recently have become involved in primary care, creating a pluralistic environment and allowing for the development of multidisciplinary primary care teams. Physician assistants and nurse practitioners emerged in the 1960s and 1970s as the "new health practitioners" and usually work under the supervision of physicians. The training of physician assistants and nurse practitioners generally lasts 18 to 24 months after they earn a bachelor's degree, and most nurse practitioners receive a master's degree in advanced practice nursing. The number of these providers has grown steadily such that there is now one primary care physician assistant or nurse practitioner for every 2.5 primary care physicians (Institute of Medicine [IOM], 1996). A recent survey by the American Academy of Family Physicians (1998) showed that the majority of its members have worked with a physician assistant or nurse practitioner. These health care professionals help physicians by seeing patients with common and less serious problems, by spending more time with patients, and by providing patient education. Primary care physicians find that working with a physician assistant or a nurse practitioner makes them more efficient and frees up their time to care for patients with more complex and serious problems (Fitzgerald, Jones, Lazar, McHugh, & Wang, 1995).

Other health professionals working with primary care physicians include clinical pharmacists, nutritionists and dieticians, physical therapists, patient educators, and mental health professionals. As mental health professionals look to integrate their work in medical settings, they would do well to look at how other professionals work with primary care physicians.

The diversity and complexity of health problems, the economics of health care (which now consumes over $1 trillion, or 15% of the gross domestic product), the diversity in numbers of health care providers, and the lack of a national health care system in the United States all result in a chaotic environment for primary care. For example, medical specialists and subspecialists, who make up two-thirds of American physicians, provide about 25% of the primary care in the United States generally in a fragmented and more expensive manner (Spiegel, Rubenstein, Scott, & Brook, 1983). In addition, about 40% of Americans seek some of their health care from "alternative providers" such as chiropractors, naturopaths, and homeopaths (Eisenberg et al., 1998). Mental health professionals in independent practices also provide a "slice" of primary care services.

A growing trend in the United States is to bring primary care together in a whole person context, with a rational system of professionals working together to provide high-quality care at a reasonable or socially affordable cost.

Definition and Nature of Primary Care

Many definitions of primary care have evolved since the term originated in the 1960s. Two pediatricians, Alpert and Charney (1973), published a monograph defining and describing the attributes of primary care as first contact care, continuity of care (responsibility for the patient over time), and coordination of comprehensive care. In 1978, the Institute of Medicine (IOM) released a report that expanded the Alpert and Charney definition to care that is accessible, comprehensive, coordinated, continuous, and accountable (IOM, 1978). This definition remained dominant until the 1990s when the need to redefine primary care became evident in the context of managed care, new organized delivery systems, and the developing role of multidisciplinary providers.

Wanting to reemphasize the dominant role for physicians in primary care, the American Academy of Family Physicians (AAFP) released the following definition in 1994.

> Primary care is that care provided by physicians specifically trained
> for and skilled in comprehensive first contact and continuing care

for persons with any undiagnosed sign, symptom, or health concern (the "undifferentiated" patient) not limited by problem origin (biological, behavioral, or social), organ system, gender, or diagnosis.

Primary care includes health promotion, disease prevention, health maintenance, counseling, patient education, diagnosis and treatment of acute and chronic illnesses in a variety of health care settings (e.g., office, inpatient, critical care, long-term care, home care, day care). Primary care is performed and managed by a personal physician, utilizing other health professionals, consultation and/or referral as appropriate.

Primary care provides patient advocacy in the health care system to accomplish cost-effective care by coordination of health care services. Primary care promotes effective doctor-patient communication and encourages the role of the patient as a partner in health care.

Acknowledging the importance of primary care physicians, but taking a much less physician-centric position, in 1996 the IOM released what is probably the most detailed study of primary care to date. The new IOM definition of primary care is: "Primary care is the provision of integrated, accessible health care services by clinicians who are accountable for addressing a large majority of personal health care needs, developing a sustained partnership with patients, and particularly in the context of family and community" (p. 1).

The term *integrated* is used to denote the provision of comprehensive, coordinated, and continuous services that provide a seamless process of care. What links the IOM definition with the AAFP definition and past definitions is the comprehensive nature of primary care addressing any health problem at any given stage of a patient's life cycle. Providers serving in a primary care context must individually or collectively take this comprehensive responsibility for care. The coordinating function acknowledges that more than one provider is necessary to deliver primary care in a modern context, and that primary care providers should work together. Continuity of care is also an essential characteristic of primary care; it means taking responsibility for patients over time. Because of this, providers working in urgent care centers and emergency departments are not providing primary care in a full context, but rather limited primary care services.

The IOM (1996) described six core attributes that make up the nature of primary care.

1. *Excellent primary care is grounded in both the biomedical and the social sciences.* Primary care endorses the biopsychosocial model of care first articulated by Engel (1977).
2. *Clinical decision making in primary care differs from that in specialty care.* When providers take responsibility for the whole person over time, clinical decision making is done in a broader context than when they are addressing only a specific disease or organ system. Hence, the patient is well served to always have a physician to provide balance with specialists in determining what the overall best course of care is. This might include refusal of what is being offered by a specialist—for example, chemotherapy or surgery in a preterminal situation.
3. *Primary care has at its core a sustained personal relationship between patient and clinician.* This relationship is paramount to primary care. In contrast, the specialist is usually more focused on the disease or organ system rather than the whole person.
4. *Primary care does not consider mental health separately from physical health.* This holistic approach reinforces item 1 above.
5. *Opportunities to promote health and prevent disease are intrinsic to primary care practice.* Primary care is not simply disease oriented but embraces prevention as a vital component.
6. *Primary care is information intensive.* At its heart, primary care involves the providing of information. Health care information available through computers will find its greatest use in the primary care setting. Such electronic access may revolutionize primary care, with more informed patients coming to primary care providers for perspective and advice. Primary care providers may become less dependent on specialists for information.

The Modern Context of Primary Care

Primary care in the United States has begun to lapse into a fragmented assortment of providers rendering pieces of care. Many Americans exercising freedom of choice, a traditional core value, prefer to take their complaints and perceived needs to whomever they want to. The pervasive use of alternative providers indicates that they do just that. Within primary care, a buffet of professionals could market their services directly to the public who try to match perceived needs. Much of this happened in the 1980s, and health care costs escalated at three times the rate of inflation, with U.S. health care expenditures in this decade alone going from $250 billion to over $900 billion (Mullen, 1998). The payors of health care, which are private businesses purchasing health insurance as an employee benefit, and the government purchasing health care for the elderly (Medicare) and those with the lowest income (Medicaid), have taken control of health care costs. Organized delivery systems formed under the euphemism of managed care, and most Americans now get their care with some restriction of choice of providers. Primary care providers, which were marginalized during the 1980s as Americans could bypass them at will, are back in the center of health care by providing first contact, comprehensive, and continuous care. As the IOM report (1996) described in detail, this is better health care for all.

In this modern context of organized systems for delivering health care to defined populations on a predetermined budget, primary care is evolving rationally. With a commitment to comprehensiveness, coordination, and efficiency (the financial element), primary care physicians are working as employees of large multispecialty groups who are increasingly employing other health professionals. This modern context of primary care holds exciting opportunities for mental health professionals.

The Practice of Primary Care

Each primary care physician is responsible for 1,500 to 3,000 patients, depending on age, severity of illness, and availability of referrals. Seniors, over the age of 65, visit the physician on average three times more than do young and middle-aged adults (AAFP, 1998). Primary care physicians willing and able to care for AIDS patients can be kept busy with 100 to 200 patients. Primary care physicians in a large group will have a larger panel of patients since access to referral specialists is readily available. Primary care physicians assuming more complete responsibility, even up to 95% of all visits, will have a smaller panel of active patients or will see a larger number of patients each day. Being in copractice with a physician assistant or nurse practitioner allows a primary care physician to assume responsibility for more patients.

A typical primary care physician sees 20 to 25 patients in the office each day, dominated by routine 10- to 15-minute office visits for acute and chronic follow-up problems. The physician will devote 30 to 60 minutes for general checkups for adults and 15 to 20 minutes for well child care and prenatal care. Primary care physicians who still perform hospital care will "make rounds" on one to five patients for about an hour in the morning before office hours. Home visits, nursing home care, new hospital admissions, committee work, and meetings often take up lunch hours and evenings. Since primary care is a 24-hour 7-day responsibility, primary care physicians take after-hour calls for their patients or in rotation with other physicians in their group. These extended hours and contin-uous demands can result in physicians' feeling ultimately responsible for patients they share with other providers who take less responsibility, either in time or in scope of services. The average work week of a primary care physician is 55 to 60 hours of direct service (AAFP, 1998).

In addition to the 20 to 25 patients seen each day, another 20 to 25 patients per physician are treated each day in the office by nurses who check blood pres-sures, refill prescriptions, handle financial matters, coordinate referrals, and give advice. Including receptionists, billing staff, and "back office" nursing staff, there are three to four employees for every provider. The primary care physician's office is a busy place!

The range of primary care services includes prevention, acute care, chronic care, and referrals (Kroenke & Mangelsdorff, 1989). Prevention, the newest area of primary care, is becoming an important part of the work. Well child care is time honored, but preventive care for adults has matured over the past two to three decades to include health promotion advice, including advice on nutrition and exercise, along with screening for early detection of disease, such as with mammograms and Pap smears. Since unhealthy lifestyles account for at least 50% of illness and premature death, health advice on lifestyle is recognized to be of paramount importance to primary care. The psychosocial dimensions and pos-sible role for mental health professionals in preventive services are tantalizing and only beginning to be considered (Fisher & Ransom, 1997).

The oldest and still most common part of primary care is acute care, which accounts for about one-third of visits. Respiratory infections and sprains and strains tend to dominate, but complex problems such as headaches, fatigue, and abdominal pain require a biopsychosocial approach. The old paradigm was to rule out all physical causes before considering the psychosocial, but more sophis-ticated primary care physicians take a holistic approach with mind-body dualism from the start.

With an aging population, chronic problems are the fastest growing part of primary care. Hypertension, diabetes, depression, anxiety disorders, arthritis, obesity, lipid disorders, and asthma are the most common and often occur together in middle-aged and older adults. Increasingly, a single provider is being seen as inadequate to manage chronic disease, and as a result, delivery systems are developing management programs with a multidisciplinary team of providers. Mental health providers could be contributing to these teams, however there is currently a lack of mental health professionals trained to work in medical settings.

Referrals are an important part of primary care. Five to 15% of patients seen are given a referral, depending on the setting and availability. Referrals to medical and surgical physician specialists are common, as are referrals to physical thera-pists, nutritionists, weight control programs, social workers, and mental health professionals. As stated elsewhere in this book, 50% or more of mental health care is provided in a primary care setting, and referrals are made for the more serious problems (Barrett, Barrett, Oxman, & Gerber, 1988; Leon et al, 1995).

It is important for mental health professionals to realize that primary care physicians will not want to have all mental health problems usurped from them as they care for the whole person (deGruy, 1997). Seamless relationships can develop, with a synergistic improvement of care by both primary care physicians and mental health providers working together in a primary care setting. The mental health professional will still be a referral provider, and his or her proxim-ity in primary care clinics allows for better detection and appreciation for mental health problems.

Because the primary care office sees the undifferentiated patient, primary care providers must learn to live with uncertainty as to the actual diagnosis, which often only becomes evident over time. Being out in the community and the entry point of health care carries both the reward of helping people and the stress of continually dealing with a great variety of biopsychosocial problems. Forming an integrated health care team, including a mental health provider, offers an oppor-tunity to more effectively address the variety and the range of human suffering in every community.

The Future of Primary Care

The practice of primary care is likely to change radically in the near future (Geyman & Hart, 1994). The office visit model of care grew out of expediency and fee-for-service reimbursement. As more health care becomes prepaid, or cap-itated, there is no financial incentive for office visits. Moreover, computers provide readier access to medical information and expand options for communi-cation. Electronic mail is more convenient for communication than the tele-phone in that both parties do not have to engage at the same time. Since much of primary care at a basic level is sharing of information, electronic methods may replace many office visits. Face-to-face contact will always be essential for most physician-patient relationships. However, in the new information environment, the primary care physician and other providers may see patients less often but be able to give them more time, both during visits and elsewhere. This may facili-tate healing practices, including attention to the whole person. More time to focus on the more complex or sicker patients will be good for primary care physi-cians and mental health professionals, especially if they are working together.

Specialty Care

Development of Specialty Care

Specialty care in medicine is as old as recorded history. Durant (1935) described how medicine in Pharaonic Egypt (3000–1500 B.C.) thrived and then declined due to specialization followed by overspecialization. The ancient Greeks fostered generalism, but the Romans preferred specialists (Durant, 1939, 1944). Henry VIII had 16 different specialists ministering to him at his death (Durant, 1956). Louis XIV cried out, "I'm dying from too many doctors!" (Durant & Ariel, 1963). With the 17th-century Age of Reason and birth of the scientific method, medical generalists and specialists flourished, the latter mainly reserved for the wealthy classes.

In the 20th century, physicians started to provide beneficial care to the patient, rather than actual harm or simply a placebo treatment (Starr, 1982). Osler (1932), regarded as the greatest American physician, heralded the start of the 20th century with a plea that all specialist physicians be first trained as good generalists. Unfortunately, as the modern university-based medical schools flourished after the Flexner Report of 1910, specialist training began right after medical school, without the benefit of a general medical background.

In the United States, most of the specialties became organized as distinct entities in the 1930s. They remained small in numbers until after World War II, when the most recent "age of specialization" began. In 1950, two-thirds of American physicians were generalists (Starr, 1982). By 1980, two-thirds were specialists, and that proportion grew to 70% by 1990 (Colwill, 1992). This trend toward specialization has occurred to a lesser degree throughout the developed world. The 1990s has seen some return to primary care, and the percentages have stabilized. Large organized delivery systems, such as Kaiser Permanente, prefer to have an equal mix of specialists and generalists or primary care physicians. As more large delivery systems with a similar mindset develop, there is a perception of an oversupply of specialists while primary care physicians are in demand.

Differences between Specialists and Primary Care Physicians

The fundamental differences between specialists and primary care physicians are the focus of responsibility and the relative degree of expertise in a given area of medicine. Ideally, any physician would place the welfare of the person first and the disease second. However, at times, specialists can see their responsibility as treating certain diseases or parts of the body, leaving the "big picture" of the person's overall life and well-being to others. Indeed, most specialists believe that their focused treatment is always for the benefit of the overall person, and it usually is. A common exception to this would be continued aggressive treatment of a cancer when the patient has become inevitably terminal.

Specialists gain their focused expertise, and departure from general medical care, through years of specialty training. Training to be a medical specialist, such as a cardiologist or gastroenterologist, involves an additional two to three years after a three-year internal medicine residency. Training in the surgical specialties generally lasts five years after medical school but may be as long as seven years, as for cardiothoracic surgery or neurosurgery. Subspecialization refers to specialty training after the physician has completed residencies in fields such as internal medicine, pediatrics, or general surgery, with the focused expertise more narrowly defined. For example, cardiology and gastroenterology are subspecialties of internal medicine, and urology and neurosurgery are subspecialties of surgery.

As summarized by Rosser (1996), "The specialist, whose focus is a disease, organ system, or investigative procedure, should provide integrated accessible health care services, but cannot address a large majority of the patient's health care needs. Nor is the specialist likely to maintain a sustained partnership with patients or to practice within the context of family and community" (p. 139). Some specialists try to provide comprehensive primary care, a so-called hidden system of primary care, but such care is more expensive and less comprehensive than care given by generalist primary care physicians (Franks & Fiscella, 1998; Rosenblatt, Hart, Baldwin, Chan, & Schneeweiss, 1998).

While the focused expertise of a specialist is highly valued and accounts for many of the benefits of modern medicine, the lack of broad general knowledge is sometimes problematic. Recently, a 77-year-old woman went to see a general physician because she had no "family doctor." Her three physicians of many years were a pulmonologist, a cardiologist, and a gastroenterologist, based on her three principal diseases. She developed a rash, and her pulmonologist suggested she see her general physician, telling her, tongue-in-cheek, that he "flunked" dermatology. After treating her simple dermatitis, the general physician determined that her three principal diseases were highly interrelated as one overall illness complex. The three specialists remained important, but the general physician's ability to integrate her care resulted in less medication and improved well-being.

One physician, who trained in obstetrics/gynecology after residency training and four years of family practice, observed a colleague in the same specialty referring a patient to a dermatologist for a rash he quickly determined to be simple poison ivy. Such examples argue for better general knowledge and skills for specialists, yet there is little evidence of this given the continuing demands of greater expertise in focused areas for specialists as reductionistic medical science and technology evolve. Hence, a rational system of health care integrates generalists with specialists.

In general, care by specialists is more expensive than primary care. The exception to this is the care for problems ordinarily requiring a specialist, for example, most cancers and serious heart disease. In such cases, a specialist can hone in on the problem with special expertise where a primary care physician may do extraneous tests or treatment. A rational system of health care has primary care providers at the entry point of care, providing services for common health problems (about 80% of care), but referring patients to or consulting with specialists when appropriate. Mental health providers can be specialists for mental health problems or provide primary mental health care. Hence, mental health providers may work in primary care environments with primary care physicians or in a specialty environment, working alone or with psychiatrists.

Specialties and Subspecialties

In an integrated health care setting, the mental health professional may work alongside specialty care providers. Therefore, it is important for the mental health care provider to have an understanding of the variety of cultures that exist within medical specialties and subspecialties.

The American Board of Medical Specialties (ABMS) recognizes 24 specialties and 76 subspecialties. (These are listed in Appendix D.) The language is confusing since primary care specialists in family practice, internal medicine, and pediatrics are also considered generalists who care for the whole person over time. Another confusion is that the distinction between a specialty and a subspecialty may be more political than rational. For example, orthopedic surgery and neurological surgery are listed as specialties rather than subspecialties of surgery. This reflects their organizations' desire for full autonomy, rather than any influence by the American College of Surgeons. In contrast, the internal medicine subspecialties have remained under the umbrella of internal medicine, which causes some confusion with the general internists who are in primary care.

As medical students learn when they try to decide on a career in medicine, each specialty seems to have its own culture. The content and culture of the most common specialties are summarized in Appendix D. The descriptions are tailored to what may be of interest to mental health professionals working in medical settings. Most medical specialists are highly biomedical in their focus, which is a result of their training. The biopsychosocial model has permeated primary care to a limited extent, but it is a rare approach in specialty care.

For the first four decades after World War II, Americans enjoyed increasing access to specialists and became accustomed to self-selecting them for their problems. Multispecialty clinics flourished, with a patient's problems listed and then categorized for triage to various corresponding specialists. Health insurance became the biggest payor of such care, and by the 1980s health care in America became very expensive and even unaffordable to those who purchased insurance. Because the government, through Medicare and Medicaid, pays for more than 40% of health care costs, it has become alarmed by open access to specialists. The managed care revolution of the 1990s has been largely one of cost control through limiting access to specialist physicians. The access-to-specialist issue has become one of great debate, with numerous state laws being passed to ensure the patient's right to choose a physician (Kassirer, 1994).

As health care systems evolve, there will be greater integration among all physicians and greater involvement of other health care professionals. Because the practice of medicine is moving more to a multispecialty group approach, with primary care and specialty providers on the same team, mental health professionals working in medical settings are likely to interact regularly with physician specialists. For this reason, it is important for mental health professionals to have an understanding of the primary and specialty care cultures. Such understanding and respect for physicians' work will go a long way toward developing collegial relationships, with better health care for patients.

The Role of Mental Health Providers in Specialty Care

Mental health providers can play a large role in specialty care, depending on the specialty and how the care delivery system is organized both operationally and financially. For example, in health psychology, a specialty in cancer (oncology) is one of the most rapidly growing fields, owing to the growing body of research on the psychosocial aspects of cancer and what interventions are most helpful to patients. Other specialty areas where there is an increasing body of literature documenting the psychosocial impacts of biomedical illnesses and biopsychosocial interventions for illnesses include infertility (obstetrics and gynecology), chronic illness and chronic pain (rheumatology), spinal cord injury (physical medicine), diabetes (endocrinology), asthma (pulmonary physicians or allergists), sexual dysfunction (urology and obstetrics/gynecology), attention deficit disorder, migraine, and Parkinson's disease (neurology).

While this body of knowledge exists, most patients are not receiving benefits from this extensive clinical knowledge, possibly owing to operational and financial constraints. We informally interviewed a neurologist, urologist, and cardiologist from one medical group about their utilization of therapists. In this group, the mental health treatment was "carved out." Not only was mental health not part of the health care group, but the physicians and therapists rarely communicated, if at all. Because they often did not know each other, an example of a physician's referral for the patient would go something like this: "The biomedical illness that you have can create some psychological symptoms. Here is a 1-800 number that you can call to get the names of three mental health professionals in your neighborhood who you can talk to about this problem. I'll see you in a month for a re-check on your problem."

As a result of this type of referral, the patient may choose a mental health provider who has no particular expertise in treating that patient's problem, who may never communicate with the patient's treating physician (except perhaps for an acknowledgment letter of the referral), and who may spend the first session searching for a *DSM-IV-TR* diagnosis that can justify payment of the session. Following the typical patient's negative experience with a referral, it is no surprise that the three specialist physicians we interviewed saw little use in "making a mental health referral." In fact, although they all reported being aware of the patient's mental health benefits, they rarely offered these benefits to their patients. They reported that their patients might (1) take offense at the referral, (2) probably wouldn't go anyway, and (3) if they did go, they would report back that it wasn't helpful.

When pressed about whether they would use the mental health professional to provide patient education about the psychosocial aspects of the illness, the three specialists who were interviewed said no. Either they would educate their patients themselves or their nurses would. Perhaps one reason why mental health services are rarely used in specialty care is that the services available have been poorly coordinated. Burgeoning mental health services in oncology may be one exception to this trend and may serve as a model for other medical specialties. Despite the fact that integrated mental health care has a great deal to offer physicians and patients in specialty care, before the burgeoning clinical knowledge can be applied, operational and financial systems must be in place to support coordinated and integrated care (see Chapter 3).

Chapter 2

The Culture and Context of Mental Health Care

What is mental health care? What are the common treatment strategies? What professional credentials must someone have to provide mental health care? These questions are not easy to answer. In fact, it is difficult to determine a common description or definition of traditional mental health care. For example, in 1985 at a historic conference sponsored by the Milton H. Erickson Foundation, recognized leaders in the field of psychotherapy gathered to share ideas and explore similarities and differences in approaches to treatment. Interestingly, the differences were so great that the organizer of the conference concluded there is no single mutually agreed-upon definition of what constitutes psychotherapy or mental health care (Zeig, 1987b).

This diversity is likely due to the varied history of the profession and the practice of mental health treatment, in addition to the fact that mental health treatment is currently characterized by divisions within the profession, in terms of both approach to treatment and professional affiliation. These differences among professionals have worsened at the macrosystem level as a result of health care reimbursement reform and the scarcity of the mental health care treatment dollar. Consequently, the current macrosystem context of mental health care is characterized by proverbial professional arm wrestling—jockeying, if you will, for positions of prominence in the mental health marketplace.

Differences among the profession and practice of mental health care are unfortunate, however, considering that research has failed to show consistent significant differences in patient outcomes across treatment approaches (Beutler,

Machado, & Neufeldt, 1994; Norcross, 1986) and across professional affiliation or training background (e.g., Doherty & Simmons, 1996). Essentially, regardless of the model of psychotherapy used or of the professional background, affiliation, or licensure of the clinician, patient outcomes have more to do with patient characteristics and the patient's relationship with the clinician than any other variable. In short, the best clinician is the best clinician regardless of professional background and training, affiliation, or licensure (Garfield, 1994; Krupnick et al., 1996).

The current culture and context of mental health care can be understood best through a discussion of the modern history of mental health treatment.

Diversity in Treatment Approaches

Although the treatment of mental health problems is at least as old as medicine and probably predates the advent of recorded history (Jackson, 1999), most consider Sigmund Freud as the founder of modern mental health treatment. In the late 1800s, Freud published his first works describing the treatment of mental health problems. It was also at this time that modern psychiatry began, with physicians beginning to specialize in the care and treatment of disorders of the mind.

Probably influenced by its European beginnings, this early psychotherapy emphasized an analysis of the past and the active influence of the past on the present (Zeig, 1987a). From this analytical tradition, it was assumed that self-reflection and careful examination of one's past led to change-promoting insight. The therapeutic relationship, with the therapist as a "blank screen" on which associations with one's past could be made, became the medium for self-understanding. Because therapy was conducted in a way that controlled for anything that would interfere with this relationship, analysts would exclude family and others from the therapy and work exclusively with the patient. Therapists standardized the length of appointments, both across sessions with the same patient and across different patients. They also treated the material disclosed within the treatment sessions with the strictest of confidentiality, including information as to whether or not the person was even being treated. Confidentiality and consistency became the hallmarks of good treatment.

Beginning in the United States in the early 1900s and gaining prominence during and immediately after World War II, psychologists began developing and promoting more pragmatic, present-focused approaches to mental health treatment (Zeig, 1987a). The humanistic approach of Carl Rogers, for example, gained in prominence at this time. Rather than emphasizing self-understanding as the goal of treatment, this approach emphasized awareness and personal experience. Self-expression and the patient's experience of the present became the focus of treatment.

As a result of a concentrated research emphasis by psychologists to better understand behavior, the behavioral and cognitive approaches to treatment began to surface shortly after the 1950s. Clinicians working from these models of therapy viewed mental health problems as the result of social conditioning and learning. The idea behind treatment was that anything that is learned can be unlearned. With this in mind, treatment focused on unlearning dysfunctional thoughts and behaviors and learning functional ones. Biofeedback and other popular methods of treatment for mental health problems were a result of this movement.

Out of the tradition of anthropology, a fourth genre of mental health treatment began in the 1960s. This tradition saw mental health problems developing as a result of a person's most important relationships. Using this treatment approach, clinicians did not see the individual patient as the unit of treatment; rather the family or couple or other relationship unit became the focus of treatment. For these clinicians the focus in treatment was what was happening between people, rather than what was happening inside individuals. Marriage and family therapy as a profession grew out of this way of treating mental health problems. More recent developments in this area have emphasized the resourcefulness of individuals and have focused on solutions to problems rather than on the problems themselves.

These four movements represent only broad characterizations of the treatment approaches currently in existence. Rollo May (1987) estimated that there are currently over 300 distinct models of therapy! While this is an incredible number of published approaches to psychotherapy, it underscores the difficulty in determining the common culture and context of mental health care.

Only recently have attempts been made to integrate approaches to treatment by focusing on common elements of successful mental health care (e.g., Norcross, 1987; Zeig, 1987b, 1995). However, these attempts to create a unifying, integrative, or eclectic approach have not been met with great success. For example, the conference mentioned earlier, sponsored by the Milton H. Erickson Foundation (Zeig, 1987a), was met with enthusiasm and judged a great success. However, a second conference, seven years later with many of the same presenters, revealed that in general the leaders in the field had not altered their approaches to treatment as a result of what they "learned" from each other during the first conference (Zeig, 1995). These leaders in the field were still espousing their same models of treatment.

As can be seen from this discussion, mental health care is based on models of treatment that have their origins in philosophy, research, and theory. Because of the appeal of these models to individual clinicians, it is difficult to arrive at a common treatment protocol or treatment approach. Treatment of a condition by one clinician may consist of 20 weekly sessions with the patient alone, while treatment of the same condition by another clinician working from another perspective may involve the entire family in four to six sessions.

The Multiplicity of Mental Health Professions

Five mental health professions are recognized by the Center for Mental Health Services of the Substance Abuse and Mental Health Services Administration (SAMHSA) as being able to provide independent mental health practice. These are psychiatry, psychiatric nursing, psychology, marriage and family therapy, and clinical social work. Licensure in most states designates clinicians in these professions as distinct and as qualified to provide mental health treatment. However, there are also a number of other mental health professions designated by titles such as mental health professional and professional counselor. Each of these "professions" has its own professional organization and licensure. In addition, each engages in its own (independent) lobbying efforts and establishes its own professional standards. In contrast, physicians, regardless of their training or specialization, belong to the American Medical Association and share the same licensure. Whereas psychologists belong to the American Psychological Association, marriage and family therapists belong to the American Association of Marriage and Family Therapy, and clinical social workers belong to the National Association of Social Workers and have their own separate licenses.

What this means is that each of these mental health disciplines competes with one another in the national and local arena for the lion's share of the elusive health care dollar. The result is an environment in which lobbying efforts designed to improve the mental health care outcomes and the quality of care unwittingly become turf battles, with one group of professionals arguing that it is more qualified or equally qualified with others to provide mental health services. However, this political posturing does not take into account the research evidence, which suggests that professional affiliation or type of license results in no significant difference in patient treatment outcome (e.g., Doherty & Simmons, 1996).

In general, two differences exist between professions. The first is that, in general, psychiatrists, as physicians, are the only mental health professionals able to prescribe medications and medical treatments. (Although there have been and continue to be noteworthy attempts by some to broaden psychopharmacology prescription powers to psychologists, these privileges have yet to be granted.) The second is that specialized training is needed to administer and interpret many, but not all, psychological tests. This specialized training is part of the standard training programs in psychology; however, it is not part of the training program in social work or marriage and family therapy. As a result, psychologists in general are licensed to administer and interpret a broad range of specialized psychological tests while licensed clinical social workers and marriage and family therapists are not.

Although our list of differences between professions is not exhaustive, it is sufficient for underscoring the fact that we see fewer differences between licensed mental health professions than similarities. Essentially, we believe that most of what therapists of all stripes do is very similar, with just a few distinct legal or professional differences. We believe that it is the culture and context of the mental health care environment that contribute to the perceived differences in professions, while real differences are difficult to determine.

Integrating Traditions of Mental Health Care with the Practice of Collaborative Care

It is often difficult at first for mental health clinicians to make the transition from the traditional independent practice model to a collaborative or team-based practice model. Nevertheless, this transition is often met with success. The difficulty appears to be in the fact that the culture and context of traditional mental health care are often in conflict with those of primary medical care.

On the surface, the differences between the two cultures are often great and, since the therapist is entering the medical territory, the therapist does most of the adapting (Patterson, Bischoff, Scherger, & Grounds, 1996). In time, physicians also change through contact with the therapists. In addition, the longer therapists practice in medical settings, the more they realize that physicians, nurses, and therapists are after the same fundamental things—best care for patients, appropriate and helpful caregiving relationships, protection of privacy, a good patient experience in the clinic, a good clinician experience in the clinic, and financial viability of the practice. Differences in culture and style recede in importance as deeper understandings about the commonalities across all clinicians begin to emerge.

Here we identify the most important cultural and contextual issues of traditional mental health care that exert the greatest impact on the practice of collaborative health care. We chose these cultural issues because of their prominent effect on the practice of psychotherapy. Most therapists, regardless of mental health profession, would be subject to the influence of these issues.

The Primacy of Confidentiality

Psychotherapists generally place great emphasis on respecting the confidentiality of patient information. Even with a signed release of information, therapists generally are reluctant to disclose all but the most minimal information about their patients and the treatment being provided. This is true even with collaborators, office mates, professional colleagues, and sometimes even clinical supervisors.

This strict guard against breaches in confidentiality probably stems from two notable influences. First, the psychoanalytical influence that has pervaded all of psychotherapy emphasizes strict confidentiality as a curative factor in psychotherapy. This tradition holds that unless patients believe that material can be shared under rules of strictest confidence, true change will not be able to take place. Under this tradition, the therapeutic relationship and the trust the patient has in the therapist are actually quite fragile. As a result, therapists are reluctant to share even the most basic of client information out of concern for breaking the foundation of trust that is so important to progress in therapy. Second, the stigma attached to mental illness and having a therapist is still quite pervasive. Therapists are aware of this stigma and so respect the confidentiality of clients. Because of both the fragility of the therapeutic relationship and the assumed stigma of receiving mental health care, strict rules of confidentiality are common in the culture of mental health care.

This approach to confidentiality is often at odds with the culture and context of the primary medical care environment. This does not mean that primary care physicians and other primary care medical professionals do not also adhere to strict guidelines with regards to confidentiality. However, there is generally an acknowledgment that information about patients must be shared with collaborating colleagues in order for the team of medical professionals to do their job. As a result, confidentiality is seen much differently in the primary care medical environment. For example, notes are written so that every treatment provider working with the patient can have access to a broad range of information about the patient. Both formal (e.g., rounds) and informal (e.g., curbside consultations) conversations about patients occur frequently without first informing the patient about exactly whom will be consulted and what information will be shared. Interruptions to medical interviews and therapy sessions are common in primary care medical facilities, contributing to the loss of confidentiality. Because of the less strict approach to confidentiality, this primary care practice environment frequently challenges the culture of traditional mental health care (see chapter 6 for more information on confidentiality in integrated medical settings).

The Responsibility for Treatment

Therapists practicing from the traditional mental health care model assume full responsibility for the mental health care treatment plan. Although patients are often seen as collaborators in the therapy process, therapists are still the ones making treatment decisions. In general, therapists believe that they need to have flexibility to make treatment decisions in the best interests of their clients, regardless of the demands of the referring agency, the family, the spouse, the courts or government, or any other entity seeking to influence the treatment.

However, when working within a primary care medical setting, it is the primary care physician, not the therapist, who is ultimately responsible for the treatment that is provided. The lack of maneuverability that accompanies this fact is difficult for many therapists to manage. However, except for a minority of cases seen within the primary care medical setting, therapists can expect to provide one part of an entire range of biopsychosocial care that is managed by the primary care physician.

Variable Length of Patient Sessions

Most mental health treatment sessions take place within a 50-minute time period. Rarely do therapists break from this standard. When they do diverge from this time period, it is usually to spend more time with a client rather than less. So, while one may encounter a therapist who schedules 80- to 90-minute sessions, it would be even rarer to find a therapist who schedules sessions every half an hour. The session is traditionally uninterrupted time with a patient, and interruptions are viewed as a disruption to the therapeutic process and a hindrance to maintaining a therapeutic relationship. The result is that most therapists will see at most six to eight clients a day. Contrast this treatment schedule with the treatment schedule of a primary care physician who sees 20 to 25 patients a day in 10-

to 15-minute sessions that are often interrupted by phone calls and knocks on the door, and the difference in treatment culture becomes glaringly obvious.

Therapists working in primary care settings are often challenged to see patients for shorter periods of time, to match the time-pressured culture of the primary care setting. However, aside from the time pressure of the office, to the extent that therapists have found a focus (with patients and as team members), they will tend to find that the work often does not take 50 minutes and will offer shorter appointments. Thus, half-hour follow-up appointments are often plenty of time for therapists to meet with patients. In addition, it is not uncommon for therapists to meet with patients in unscheduled visits or for a few minutes before or after patients' appointments with physicians. Therapists working in a primary care office will often continue to see clients in 50-minute sessions; however, many different formats are possible and can be expected within these settings.

The Time-limited Nature of Treatment

Similar to specialty care in medicine, traditional mental health care is provided on a time-limited basis. Treatment may entail several weeks or several years of therapy sessions, and although the therapist and patient may address multiple problems or life issues over the course of treatment, therapy has a distinct ending. Once therapy is completed, patients may return for additional treatment, but typically a problem must be identified in order for treatment to be re-started. The mental health care contract is by its nature problem-determined.

Primary medical care, however, emphasizes a continuation in care through both periods of overt medical need and routine health maintenance. Although the treatment of specific conditions may have a distinct beginning and ending, treatment of the patient in primary care is ongoing. In fact, patients are encouraged to schedule annual check-ups and to access other primary care medical services in times of wellness.

This difference in how care is conceptualized is difficult for many therapists to incorporate into their practice. For many, when a subsequent session is not scheduled, the file on the patient is closed. However, in a primary care medical facility, the file is left open indefinitely (given the stability of health care insurance, patient mobility, and other factors). The primary care physician and the corresponding team of biopsychosocial health care providers are on call to provide ongoing health care for the patient, whether it is for a diagnosable condition or routine maintenance of health.

The time-limited nature of mental health treatment is also reinforced by common third party reimbursement of service policies. Although differences in reimbursement procedures will be described in more detail later in this chapter, it is important to point out that most mental health coverage specifies a limited number of outpatient mental health sessions per year (e.g., 20 sessions per insured member). In order for therapists to be reimbursed under these policies, each mental health visit must typically be justified with the identification of a mental health problem. Unlike primary medical care, there is no reimbursement category for annual check-up or periodic wellness interview.

Theory-based Approaches to Treatment

Traditionally, psychotherapy is informed more by theory than by the results of research. Therapists have theories about the development of psychopathology and other problems and how to conduct treatment for these problems. The operation of treatment strategies and techniques (i.e., what happens in therapy) and treatment plans are best explained theoretically. Thus, therapists use an elaborate theoretical language to communicate with one another about the psychology of their patients' problems and the treatment they are providing. This language and way of talking about patients and problems is part of the psychotherapeutic culture. Therapists, even those from differing theoretical backgrounds, understand one another and appreciate communication according to theoretical principles.

In comparison, primary care physicians take a less theoretical and a more evidence-based approach to medicine. Treatment protocols, medications, and medical procedures typically undergo careful empirical scrutiny before becoming part of the mainstream of clinical practice in medicine. However, this has not been the case with mental health care. In fact, most approaches to psychotherapy, complete with their treatment protocols, have not been subjected to empirical investigation of their outcomes or the processes occurring within the therapies that make them successful. This disparity in practice strategies between medicine with its evidence-based approach and psychotherapy with its theory-based approach often inhibits successful integration.

Not only does this disparity affect the use of treatment protocols, but also it affects the type of information that informs treatment decisions. For example, in evidence-based medicine, physicians look for the presence of symptoms that have been identified through empirical study to indicate a specified medical condition. However, psychotherapists often rely on intuition and hypothesis testing to determine treatment direction. Theory, clinical experience, and therapist biases are used to inform these hypotheses. The closest guide to assessment and treatment that the field of mental health has to evidence-based medicine is the *DSM-IV-TR* published by the American Psychiatric Association (2000).

On the other hand, this is not to say that physicians do not rely on intuition, clinical experience, and anecdotal evidence when making clinical decisions. Physicians do use these other resources, but the evidence-based approach to medicine is prominent within the field and gaining momentum, especially in training programs. Evidence-based medicine means that when making clinical decisions, the practitioner considers all the available information, especially that derived from research, on the effectiveness of a course of treatment, including related health outcomes (Handley & Stuart, 1994). Evidence-based medicine carefully considers the research literature and uses it to guide clinical decision making. The goal of this approach to medicine is to improve health outcomes (Clancy & Kamerow, 1996; Handley & Stuart, 1994).

Because the theoretical language and theoretically informed treatments of mental health care are often so different from the approach taken by physicians, a communication and treatment barrier exists between therapists and physicians. Our experience has been that while therapists working in primary care settings need to continue to conduct treatment from a theoretical position, physicians generally are not interested in the theoretical descriptions of patient problems and treatments. Communications about treatments and patients generally are most productive when patient behaviors and interactions are emphasized, rather than why patients behave or interact as they do. This type of communication more closely matches the action-oriented, evidence-based communications of the medical environment.

Reimbursement of Services

In today's health care setting, a mental health therapist can be reimbursed in various ways. Some reimbursement systems reflect the integrated nature of the collaborative care model, whereas others do not. It is important to note that the reimbursement system is changing rapidly and varies by region. Even within particular health care settings, the policy for reimbursement is changing over relatively short periods of time. For example, in one health care setting, reimbursement went from 100% capitation to less than 40% capitation over about a 10-year period.

It is important for therapists to be aware that there are multiple ways of being reimbursed and that this should be negotiated up front. However, therapists working in the medical setting should also be aware of contextual and systemic factors that influence whether or not a particular type of reimbursement is possible. For example, therapists expect to get reimbursed for each session, yet therapy occurring within a definable session only makes up a small portion of the work they do in the primary care environment. Insurance companies struggle with how to reimburse for the care provided by mental health providers in these environments because no coding system currently exists for identifying all the work that a therapist does and how much it is worth. Physicians also find themselves in similar situations, such that they find it difficult to identify how reimbursement of mental health services should occur.

These differences in the reimbursement of services can also be confusing for patients. For example, it is not uncommon for a patient's health care plan to require a different copayment amount for medical care than for mental health care. It is not uncommon for a patient who is accustomed to a $10 copayment for an office visit to a physician to be surprised to learn that the session with the therapist working from the same office requires a copayment amount of $35 or more. This can be even more confusing when the patient is also responsible for a percentage of the mental health fee or when the mental health coverage requires that a separate deductible be met.

It is our observation that, as a result of the discrepancy of copayments and other factors (e.g., the time-limited nature of mental health treatment, the overall cost of care, reluctance to provide insurance companies with a record of mental health treatments), patients are more willing to bypass insurance to obtain mental health care than they are to bypass insurance to obtain medical care. For instance, we have had patients who, due to a change in insurance carriers, have had to change physicians because their current physician is no longer a provider within their new plan. While they have complained about needing to change physicians, they have nevertheless made the change. However, many of these patients have also requested that they be able to continue to see the mental health provider that is part of the old clinic even though that provider is not part of the new panel of providers. This request is made even though seeing the therapist would come at a greater financial cost to them than if they changed therapists.

Chapter 3

Bringing other Cultures Together: Harmonizing the Clinical, Operational, and Financial Perspectives of Health Care

Living in a World of Multiple Perspectives

Health care is full of different people with a variety of perspectives, interests, professions, and skills. The challenge is for this diverse assembly of health care professionals to integrate their work on behalf of patients and on behalf of reform of the health care environment in which they are all working (Halvorson, 1993; Miller & Luft, 1994, 1997; Rodnick & O'Connor, 1997; Shortell, Gillies, & Anderson, 1994; Sobel, 1995, 1997).

Better integration of the work of mental health professionals and physicians is the cornerstone of this book, but the larger picture of integration and collaboration needed in health care goes far beyond this. All mental health clinicians new to general health care settings need to recognize these multiple perspectives and collaborative challenges and then do what they can to navigate them effectively in their daily work, and thus promote harmony rather than conflict.

Because of the variety of caregivers in the medical setting, therapists can expect to encounter a variety of different ideas in their clinical practice (Haber & Mitchell, 1998; Starfield, 1991). With these influences come different opinions and perspectives. Usually mental health clinicians think about their own influence in their clinical practice; however, in integrated health care, they need to look at the situation from several different vantage points, as illustrated in the following case example.

For the last six weeks, Mr. Jones has been treated for a back strain caused by shoveling snow. He would like to improve; therefore, he continues to call his physician because the back pain has persisted and he feels that his needs are not being adequately met.

Dr. Williams expects Mr. Jones to be significantly improved, since the patient has completed acute care treatment for his back. The physician wants Mr. Jones to continue the recommended back exercises and to gradually discontinue his medication. He wants Mr. Jones to stop calling and to stop scheduling more visits as these do not provide any additional information and serve no apparently useful purpose.

Ms. Jasper, the clinic receptionist, would like Mr. Jones to decrease his calls and visits to the clinic because it is leading to appointment backlog and unhappiness for Dr. Williams, clinic nurses, and other patients who have more serious problems and are not able to get an appointment quickly.

Acme Health, Mr. Jones's health plan, wants Dr. Williams to stop using so many resources on a patient's condition, in this case, Mr. Jones's back, that should be significantly improved by now.

Mr. Jiggs, the clinic administrator, would like Dr. Williams and his colleagues to satisfy the health plan's wish to conserve resources in situations like this. As a result of doing so, the clinic's negotiating and financial position with the health plan would improve, in addition to the practice's ability to keep its patients and stay solvent.

Mr. Jones's wife says she is "worn out" and wants Dr. Williams to "do something" with her husband to improve his physical health as well as his recent irritable mood.

Mr. Jones's employer is indicating to Mr. Jones and Dr. Williams that employability is a possible question unless Mr. Jones reduces the amount of sick time that he is taking and his health and work performance improve.

The clinic's quality improvement committee wants Dr. Williams to follow newly developed protocols for treating low back strain, which includes attention to possible mental health factors since Mr. Jones has not recovered yet.

Ms. Carrol, the clinic's behavioral health professional, wants to help Mr. Jones (and his doctor) with his pattern of developing somatic symptoms. However, she knows that this challenge may result in more, rather than fewer, visits in the short term. Currently Mr. Jones's symptoms are the main way that he expresses significant personal distress or asks for help. Mr. Jones wants to feel better, yet he is feeling increasingly desperate and worried because he is still experiencing back pain. He also senses the growing expectation (and impatience) from everyone around him to comply, recover, "shape up," and get back to his life. As a result, Ms. Carrol is looking for ways to engage Mr. Jones in recovery in a way that satisfies the patient as well as the variety of other caregivers, especially those that are ultimately important to Mr. Jones, such as his wife and employer.

Each person involved in the system has a unique perspective, and the mental health care clinician needs to be aware of the various opinions. Ultimately, these various viewpoints suggest what treatment options are available to the patients so that they can receive the care they need.

In addition to the variety of opinions and ideas found in the medical setting, therapists can expect to encounter the following multiple perspectives in clinical practice:

- mental health practice and culture versus medical practice and culture
- patient responsibility, control, and choice versus clinician control and belief in "what is best for patients"
- individual clinician autonomy versus team accountability, collaborative practices, and organizational authority
- different practice models (e.g., academic, managed care, small specialty group practices, large integrated medical group practices)
- the obligations of provider, patient, family, school, court, lawyer, insurer, public agency, public policy maker
- technical quality versus service quality
- available science and evidence-based practice versus the continuing need to act when the science is incomplete
- clinical, operational, and financial perspectives; values and priorities in the design and management of health care systems

Health care today is not just a clinical challenge. All practices or care systems, regardless of size, complexity, or type, face three simultaneous challenges: (1) the clinical challenge of excellent patient care; (2) the operational challenge of employing efficient, well-integrated, and patient-friendly systems of care; and (3) the financial challenge of staying financially solvent, thus utilizing limited health care resources (Goetzel et al., 1998).

Better integration of traditionally separate and parallel medical and behavioral health care is just one of many ways to improve clinical care, service, and resource stewardship. Unfortunately, these clinical, operational, and financial perspectives, as well as the people who represent them, often compete rather than cooperate with one another. As a result, clashes between clinical and financial perspectives are among the most visible and destructive features of health care today. Behavioral health professionals entering medical settings will need to understand how to constructively balance financial and clinical tensions.

A conceptual model called the "three-world view" is described in this chapter to help behavioral health professionals turn such battles into constructive tensions and complementarities. All professionals entering the medical arena should, in their own way, become part of the effort to transform health care and keep tensions between clinical, operational, and financial matters from turning into battles.

"War of the Worlds": Tension between Clinical, Operational, and Financial Priorities

Discussions about redesigning health care, even at a local clinic level, are often laced with tension between clinical, administrative, and financial priorities. The goals of care, operational, and administrative systems and sound business practices are often seen as separate worlds that coexist in a fragile and uneasy peace, with occasional outbreaks that feel like the "war of the worlds."

Quality care and sound financial performance are sometimes positioned as opposing values held by opposing parties, as if improved quality automatically means higher cost, and that cost consciousness automatically means compromised quality. Most people have read about or experienced horror stories in which financial motives have compromised health care or runaway health costs have led families to financial ruin. Many people think health care has degenerated to "just a business." They see managed care as merely managed cost and the corporatization of health care as a threat to professional integrity and to quality care. Clinicians may ask themselves, "Do I have a place with integrity in this new world?" and patients may ask themselves, "Will my health plan come through for me and my family when the chips are down, or will they try to save a buck at my expense?" Those are serious questions. Health care today, on national and local levels, is overflowing with tensions between the clinical and business perspectives.

Behavioral health professionals entering medical settings should expect to encounter and constructively help to resolve such disharmony. The challenge is to help people who are trying to improve patient care and the practice environment by combining clinical, administrative, and financial perspectives and priorities into workable plans and actions. Failure to harmonize clinical, operational, and financial aspects of plans and action frequently result in the following problems and setbacks:

- a great clinical idea that died for lack of a well-supported implementation or "operational" plan
- a promising clinical improvement shelved for lack of a practical and shared view on how to cover its cost
- a new operational system or administrative procedure or technology that failed because it did not actually support the clinical process
- clinic systems, operations, and procedures that became more and more cumbersome, inefficient, and "patched together" as new demands were piled on old systems
- a new method for "improving clinician productivity" that engendered clinician resistance instead
- cost-control strategies that were viewed as a threat to quality care and professional autonomy
- "red ink" that led to closing a practice and disrupting hundreds of physician-patient relationships
- tension among people trained primarily in clinical, administrative, and financial matters
- difficult meetings in which every issue brings out simmering and personalized struggles between competing clinical, operational, and financial priorities of the practice

When conflicts of this kind are allowed to simmer, they can become chronic and take a painful course in which people become increasingly defensive. For example, clinicians may experience numbers, accounting, operational, and systems talk as intrusive, incomplete, or irrelevant to their efforts and values on behalf of patients, or that their efforts are being expressed by "production" numbers alone. At the same time, clinic systems experts may feel that they are being told by clinicians that operating procedures are rigid, bureaucratic, or a "barrier to the ineffable art of healing." Accountants and insurance professionals may feel they are being told by clinicians that "bean counting" is not the object when it comes to human health or is relevant only when it comes to correctly computing clinicians' paychecks.

Then such arguments ensue: "I thought this was a health care facility, not just a business" vs. "You clinicians just don't understand what it takes to run a health care system." "This may be a good idea, but who is going to pay for it? You clinicians have to pay much more attention to the cost of care if you expect to keep getting paid well" vs. "Who is watching out for the patient in this new world?" Almost all health care professionals have similar stories to tell.

There are no simple answers for the difficult questions and trade-offs in health care today. Much of the interpersonal and organizational tension that results from tackling these issues is unnecessary. For example, unnecessary tension results when the clinical, operational, and financial perspectives (and the people who champion them) are allowed to push each other around as if in a political struggle between adversarial parties. The key is to shift the mindset from politics to principles of good design.

This shift is critical because struggles within a practice often become politicized, bringing into play who owns the practice, who takes the financial risk, and who manages what. Although important structural features of a care system, who owns the assets, takes the risk, or is the boss makes little difference when it comes to designing an effective care system. This provocative but supportable statement is intended to shift the mindset from who has the power to principles of good design. A practical tool for doing this is developed next (Peek, 1988; Peek & Heinrich, 1995; Putman, 1990).

The Three-World View

Health care systems operate simultaneously in three worlds: clinical, operational, and financial. The following analogy illustrates how these worlds are actually simultaneous views of a health care practice or organization: An architect of a building must draw a front view, a side view, and a top view of his or her design in sufficient detail if he or she expects builders to actually build it. Without any one of these views of the building, the picture is incomplete and fabrication cannot take place. From a designer's perspective, a very similar thing holds true for health care. In this case the front view, side view, and top view are the clinical, operational, and financial views. Without drawing all three views, there is no hope of building a successful health care organization.

The clinical, operational, and financial views are called worlds here because people trained in one discipline so often experience these as separate, disparate, or even "foreign" worlds whose populations speak different languages, ask different questions, seek different outcomes, and employ different values and principles. This sense of the foreign easily begets tension, suspicion, and misunderstanding between people trained and working primarily in one of these worlds. This kind of tension between disparate worlds occurs in all kinds of organizations, not just in health care (Putman, 1990). However, in health care, it is the disparate clinical, operational, and financial worlds that need to be harmonized (Peek, 1988).

To return to the analogy, the worlds of an organization are related in the same way that the different architectural drawings of the same building are related. Taken together the three worlds represent the whole organization as viewed from key perspectives. No one of these views is the complete view, any more than any one of the perspective drawings shows the whole building or any one eyewitness account reflects what really happened (paraphrased from Putman, 1990).

The key to harmonizing disparate worlds is to display them in the same picture, just as an architect displays all three views of a building in one set of plans so one can look back and forth between the views as it is constructed. In this case, we are not showing actual care system "construction plans" (these are up to each care system to draw for itself). Instead, we show the language and logic of the clinical, operational, and financial worlds in a way that highlights their differences and commonalities, and the translations between them. If care system designers draw their actual construction plans in a way that satisfies the demands of all three worlds as shown in Table 3.1, the plans have a chance to succeed. In this sense, the three-world view is a standard for drawing "buildable" plans.

The basic lesson here is that any health care organization, program, or action must make good sense when viewed through clinical, operational, and financial lenses. No one perspective, language, or individual should be allowed to trump or subordinate the others. All action is premature until it can be shown to satisfy the requirements of the clinical, operational, and financial worlds, including relevant principles belonging to each world. This is not easy to do, but nothing less will work.

A hallmark of sound health care organization design and "managed care gone right" is that it meets these requirements. Table 3.1 simply shows the correspondences between the three views. Rather than including detailed instructions on

Table 3.1
The Three Simultaneous Worlds of a Health Care Organization

	CLINICAL	OPERATIONAL	FINANCIAL
Basic questions	What care is called for?	What will it take to accomplish care?	How will care utilize resources?
	Is it high quality?	Is it well executed?	Is it a good value?
Object	Unfolding cases and population health.	Systems	Numbers
Process	Actions	Operations	Accounting
Outcome	Achievement of health goals	Production	Bottom line
Standard	Quality and elegance	Efficiency and facility	Price and value
Relationship	Clinician-patient	Provider-customer	Vendor-buyer
Relevant principles	Ethics, science, and healing	Process and system improvement	Business and financial return

Adapted and expanded from Peek, 1988; Peek & Heinrich, 1995; Putman, 1990.

how to use this model or supplying lots of examples, we leave it to the readers to apply the principles where needed.

A key aspect of this perspective is to encourage health care professionals to use the three-world view as a means of preventing internal struggles over which world is real or which world should subordinate the others (the war of the worlds). Behavioral health clinicians entering any health care setting most likely will be exposed to three-world tensions as they become involved in planning and redesigning a care system. Behavioral health professionals should take opportunities to help harmonize the clinical, operational, and financial perspectives wherever they encounter them. Here are a few pointers.

1. Respect that the clinical, operational, and financial worlds each have their own internal logic and language. For example:

- In the clinical world people talk about care plans and clinical action with patients and families. Clinical world questions are about quality and the achievement of good outcomes and health goals.
- In the operational world, people talk about the operations and systems needed to produce services. The goals are productivity, execution, efficiency, and facility.
- In the financial world, people are concerned with utilizing care resources and with value. People talk about business goals, business processes, and accounting using numbers. The goals are a positive bottom line, the right price, and a good value.

2. Expect to hear these languages. (and don't try to make people talk just in your language). The same underlying topics can be translated from one world to another. For example, take the term productivity, which often provokes clinicians. Clinicians react because productivity is from the language system of the operational world. However there is a corresponding term in the clinical world, namely, *achievement*. Clinicians are happy to improve the achievement of health goals; they just don't like to be told to improve their productivity or the bottom line, as if it were the only reality. As this example illustrates, achievement, production, and bottom line are from the same underlying reality but are expressed differently in each language. Here is another example of a translation between languages of the three worlds.

- The clinical world's goals are quality and elegance.
- The operational world goals are efficiency and facility.
- The financial world goals are the right price and good value.

There is no conflict among these goals. Topics can be discussed alternately in different languages just as the same feature of a building is drawn alternately in different views of an architectural plan. Dialog should continue until solutions that advance the goals of all three worlds are found. It is possible.

3. *Learn about each other's worlds and languages but don't expect everyone to be experts in all three worlds.* Each person is hired for his or her expertise in one of the worlds, which is their "native language" or "dominant perspective." Clinicians are hired for their clinical skills; administrators, for their systems skills; and accountants and business managers for their financial skills. Everyone, especially leaders and managers, needs to be able to shift perspectives from one world to another, using the logic and languages of all three. It is too much to expect everyone to become an expert on everything, but it is not too much to expect people to learn enough about another person's world to appreciate its goals and methods and to treat it respectfully.

4. *If an action fails to meet the requirements of one world, it will ultimately fail in all three.* To be successful, all actions and designs have to satisfy the demands of all three worlds.

- If a program, project, or action fails clinically, it obviously fails.
- If a program fails operationally, it fails too because only programs or actions that can be implemented can achieve any clinical goals.
- If a program or an action fails to satisfy the demands of the financial world, it fails eventually. This occurs by either misallocating resources, failing to secure necessary resources, failing to make proper business arrangements with the beneficiaries of the program, or by running the organization as a whole into insolvency.

The criterion for a successful action of any kind is a satisfactory accounting in all three worlds. Any project, program, or action without a three-world analysis is not ready for prime time. Any project without a three-world view should not move forward. Back to the earlier analogy: Imagine the engineering drawings (top view, side view, and front view) of a mechanical part on its way to being manufactured. If any one of these drawings is missing or wrong, it will be impossible to manufacture the piece or it will malfunction once manufactured. The clinical, operational, and financial aspects of a health care plan need to be drawn so that they *cooperate* rather than *clash*. All clashes between clinical, operational, and financial parts should be resolved before the plan is sent to production.

5. *Never allow one world to trump the others.* Taking a three-world view means that all perspectives (clinical, operational, and financial) are honored, and no

one of them is allowed to subordinate or overpower the others. They each receive due time and due process. This important stance is starkly realistic in a practical sense and surprisingly effective in a human sense. It establishes a prime ground rule for dialog and project planning during difficult times. The three-world view should be treated as a fundamental principle for health care redesign. Like a law of nature, it isn't true because we said so, but because (like gravity) it exerts its influence whether you believe in it or not, no matter who you are.

6. *Let the three-world view remind everyone that in a profound sense it really doesn't matter who owns the assets, has the power, or is entitled to call the shots in the practice.* Effective action means satisfying the requirements of all three worlds, the fundamental criterion for good design in health care. Using one's power or authority merely to prevail or subordinate other perspectives and the people who champion them is self-defeating. Instead, good leaders use their power and authority to ensure that all action is informed by a three-world view, and that no one is allowed to push any one of the worlds off the map. Leadership and the three-world view are used to shift the nature of challenging discourse from who has the power to what is the best design.

7. *Use the three-world view to help keep peace and move forward at meetings and in communication.* If everyone realizes that those who run the meetings insist on a three-world analysis, everyone will understand that tough topics will be discussed alternately in clinical, operational, and financial terms. When using this approach, no one will become alarmed when the discussion starts off or veers off one way or another. Sometimes, clinicians panic when discussions start to employ words like "bottom line," "profit," "price," "buyer," or "customer" because they fear the clinical perspective will be pushed off the table. Because a credible financial plan is essential to the success of any clinical idea, therapists should expect that at certain times, the most intense effort will be focused in one or another of the worlds. For example, if the practice is insolvent, everyone can expect plenty of financial dialog. If quality concerns appear, everyone can expect plenty of clinical talk. Even at times of preoccupation with one of the worlds, it remains important to retain a three-world view, keeping all of them on the map and balanced in the long run.

8. *Use the three-world view as a "preflight checklist" to make sure the plan will have a chance to actually fly upon launching.* Not doing this invites waste and rework attributable to action that worked well in one world but failed to meet the demands of the others.

The consequences of failing to effectively take a three-world view are serious. First of all, the familiar tensions, battles, interpersonal struggles, or resignation will remain or intensify, along with a higher risk of failing to move forward.

Human and financial energy will be at risk from internal struggle at just the time it is needed for patient care. Beyond these familiar consequences of failing to take the three-world view, a health care organization design that gives short shrift to one of the worlds leads to predictable results.

- If the clinical world gets subordinated by the financial world, the result will likely be seen as bad managed care, for example, when care decisions or relationships with patients or insurers appear to be influenced by financial goals of owners or investors, or when clinical leadership or clinical priorities are not well integrated into overall goals and planning processes.
- If the financial world gets submerged, going out of business is the likely result. This can lead to thousands of disrupted patient-clinician relationships and carefully constructed care plans, not to mention the loss of jobs and perhaps highly developed working relationships between clinicians and staff. Limited financial expertise or interest among practice leaders, or a limited sense of "ownership" among clinicians and staff can reduce the quality of the financial world view.
- If the operational world is allowed to be subdued by the others, operating systems such as scheduling, billing, medical records, dictation, and communication can become overloaded and ultimately fail to meet demands.

The mission of the health care organization sets an internal standard for constructing and balancing the three worlds. Although success in any organization requires that the three worlds never be allowed to subordinate each other, the standards for overall success tend to be linked to the deepest purposes of the organization. For example, organizations whose history and mission are to deliver care and improve the health of the community as a public service may regard financial success only as a means to invest in necessary improvements and stay in existence for the community. On the other hand, organizations whose history and deepest mission comes from being a business corporation that makes money for owners, partners, or investors will likely have different standards for financial performance, how its financial world is constructed, and how margin is distributed or invested.

All credible health care organizations must share some baseline standard for quality care as defined primarily by the medical community, but different organizations (and the communities in which they are embedded) have different aspirations and expectations for performance that reach above this baseline. How the three worlds are balanced is affected by considerations of history, missions, and public expectations. Clinicians entering health care organizations attempting to help resolve three-world tensions will be more effective if they understand the history and particular balance the organization is trying to achieve in addition to knowing what the organization stands for and is designed to accomplish. Ultimately, therapists will be more effective at balancing the three worlds in practice if their own professional and personal values and purposes are matched well with those of the organization that they work in.

Part II
How to Build the New Profession and Practices of Collaborative Medical Care

Chapter 4

Getting Started: Bringing Mental Health into Primary Care

No matter how the opportunity to work in a medical setting may present itself, it is helpful to have practical, ready-at-hand ways to engage physicians and administrators and to navigate the unfamiliar terrain of clinics and complex care systems. The initial contacts and meetings are critical to both developing and enacting a collaborative relationship. Without such a foundation, it is unlikely that good intentions alone will survive the waning of initial enthusiasm in the face of hard work developing and supporting novel clinical, operational, and financial ways of delivering care.

In this chapter, we provide the about-to-be-integrated mental health professional with some practical approaches culled and harvested from 15 years of successes as well as failures in collaborations with medical providers, clinics, and integrated care delivery systems. Although other ways of bringing mental health into the primary care settings may exist, the consulting process that is described here is one that we found to be very useful.

A Good Time for Developing Integrated Care Practices

It is a particularly good time for mental health professionals to work in medical settings. A confluence of economics, research and need felt by primary care physicians make this a good time to develop integrated care practices. Economic forces driving cost-efficient care delivery, and health care industry trends (such as lifestyle management and more effective management of chronic ill-nesses) define the importance of integrating the mental health professional into primary care practice. O'Connor, Solberg, and Baird (1998) and deGruy (1997) described the current and future reality of primary care practice, from adding population management strategies (health maintenance, prevention of illness, and proactive management of chronic illness) to providing acute care and managing chronic illness. This enhanced primary care model addresses care delivery challenges and makes a strong conceptual case to integrate the mental health professional as one of the long missing members of the primary care team.

The research literature on the epidemiology and treatment outcomes of mental disorders treated in primary care also supports an expanded role for col-laborative comanagement and integrated, on-site behavioral health care delivery (refer to the Introduction, as well as Blount, 1998). The substantive findings of the past 20 years document the prevalence of mental disorders and subthreshold conditions in primary care that will never be referred nor reach specialty behav-ioral health. Therefore, novel organizational approaches are required to bring services to the patients. This literature also highlights the enhanced outcomes that can be achieved with collaborative primary care in behavioral health prac-tice, and the potential cost savings by addressing problems in the primary care setting (Cummings, Cummings, & Johnson, 1997).

In our experience, there is not only a need for more mental health profes-sionals to work in primary care settings but also a shortage of professionals to meet that demand. This is particularly true in smaller primary care practices, such as those in small towns or rural settings. These small primary care practices have a long-standing need for consultation and collaboration in managing the behavioral health needs of their patients.

A Consulting Process to Developing Integrated Care Placements: The Five-Stage Model

In the Intrduction, we discussed the fragmentation of care and the dissatisfac-tions experienced by physicians, patients, family members, and purchasers of care, caused by separate and parallel systems of medical and mental health care delivery. Because this legacy of separate and parallel systems affects each clinic or care delivery system in unique ways, there are no simple off-the-shelf or one-size-fits-all solutions.

As opportunities for integrated practice present themselves, a consulting approach to develop customized solutions as well as maturing the collaboration has been helpful. Using this approach, the mental health professional engages the physicians, clinic, or care system determining the local variations and specific ways that an integrated practice could be beneficial.

The consulting process outlined here can be a useful model for the therapist to use when structuring conversations of purpose, role, and clinical targets. A therapist can gradually move toward more formal planning by keeping succinct notes and volunteering to help coordinate people as needed. In all cases, collaborative planning is a goal for collaborative care.

The consulting process parallels the clinical care process, which involves: (1) recognition of the problems; (2) engagement of clients as coequal participants in addressing their problems; (3) evaluation of the problem(s) through formal and informal qualitative and quantitative assessment methods; (4) management (treatment) plan—goals to focus on and steps to achieve these goals; and (5) a maintenance and follow-up plan. In the consulting process, the mental health professional uses his or her consulting role to facilitate the clinic's ability to recognize and identify problems within the current system of separate and parallel systems of medical and behavioral health care delivery (1), and to engage the clinic's leaders and physicians in assessing their readiness to change current practices in order to address the problems (2). If there is sufficient interest in developing an integrated care practice, the mental health professional facilitates an evaluation of the specific needs of the clinic's patient population (3). If the earlier steps are fruitful, then the process leads to a mutually developed management plan at the clinic level that introduces and integrates the mental health professional into the practice (office space, methods of referring and scheduling patients, integration of transcription and chart notes, financing) (4) and an ongoing maintenance plan (monitoring and performance) to ensure continued development in the desired direction (continuous quality improvement) (5) (see Table 4.1).

In the rest of this chapter, we expand on and discuss in detail these five stages of the consulting process.

Overview Questions

It is often practical to launch and guide the consultation process by posing a series of questions.

Facilitating the recognition of the problem and engaging the clients as coequal participants:
1. What important recurring problems or dissatisfactions with the psychosocial aspect of care is the clinic experiencing?
2. What kind of preferred future care vis-à-vis behavioral health would the clinic or physicians like?

Table 4.1
A Five-Stage Model of the Clinical Care Process and an
Integrated Care Clinic Consultation Process*

	THE CLINICAL CARE PROCESS	THE INTEGRATED CARE CONSULTATION PROCESS
Recognition	Patient recognizes a problem and seeks professional help to resolve it.	Clinic recognizes problems with separate and parallel systems of care delivery and seeks an integrated care solution.
Engagement	Mental health professional actively listens (appeals to what matters by paraphrasing, clarifying, and identifying) to patient's concerns.	Mental health professional facilitates discussion of problems with separate and parallel systems within the clinic (what matters to the clinic's physicians and leaders).
Evaluation	Mental health professional assesses patient's problem using formal and informal qualitative and quantitative assessments.	Mental health professional facilitates description of the clinic population in useful statistical terms and the problems appropriate for an integrated care practice within the clinic.
Management	Mental health professional negotiates with the patient specific treatment goals and steps to achieve goals.	Mental health professional facilitates an implementation team to develop clinical, operational, and and financial solutions to support integrated care practice in the clinic.
Maintenance	Mental health professional and patient develop maintenance and long-term follow-up plan.	Implementation team meets regularly to monitor and evaluate integrated care and system improvements.

*Adapted from The DIAMOND Project, 1998. The DIAMOND Project, "Depression Is A Manageable Disease," is a study of the feasibility of systematizing primary care for treatment of depression by HealthPartners Research Foundation. Funded by MacArthur Foundation. L. I. Solberg (principal investigator), L. R. Fischer (coprincipal investigator), T. F. Davis, D. S. Alter, M. A. Baird, R. L. Heinrich, S. F. Lucas, C. J. Peek, and R. P. Power

Evaluating the problems:

3. What should the clinic find out about its patient population before selecting a focus for integration?
4. To start somewhere, what should the first integration project focus on and demonstrate?
5. What type of help from behavioral health care clinicians does the clinic think it needs?

Management plan:

6. How do behavioral health providers need to be prepared for roles in the clinic?
7. How will the mental health professional be introduced and integrated into the clinic and who needs to be part of the implementation effort?
8. How will the clinic learn enough to decide whether and how to move its pilot project toward a mainstream effort?
9. What amount of mental health professional time will be needed to support a clinic-wide or mainstream effort and how will it be financed?

Helping the clinic begin to answer these questions brings the integrated practice project and its goals into sharper focus, and moves it from "ideology," "another good idea," or a "should" to a framework that truly engages the professionals involved.

Stages 1 and 2: Recognition and Engagement (Factors that Matter to Primary Care Physicians and Clinics)

In initiating discussions with primary care physicians and medical clinics, the mental health professional should engage them by focusing on *what matters*. Asking about dissatisfactions with separate and parallel systems of medical and behavioral health care delivery in clinical practice will provide valuable information and discussion. In our experience, there are recurring themes of dissatisfaction that occur locally, regionally, and nationally. Clearly, improving quality and service is a priority. The purpose of early discussions is to articulate one or more practical goals for which behavioral health integration can be part of the proposed solution. Underlying these goals are common focal areas that represent a potential starting point for behavioral health care integration:

- Reduce "thick charts" reflecting somatization and high and unfocused utilization of health care resources.

- Develop effective management strategies for difficult patients who are emotionally draining to physicians and clinic staff.
- Reduce unnecessary patient visits that reduce availability of physicians.
- Develop an alternative to the problems of traditional behavioral health referrals.
- Enhance medical clinic triage of behavioral health disorders and improved consultation over medications and psychiatric emergencies.
- Reduce unnecessary hospital and referral costs.
- Promote healthy behavior for patients with chronic illnesses or risk factors.
- Help physicians manage patients with a particular disease or condition (e.g., depression, chronic pain, industrial injury).

A problem area of focus and a readiness to collaborate can be readily elicited or determined from the physicians' daily clinical experience. Attention can be directed to their experiences through the following questions:

- Have you noticed that when certain patients' names appear on your schedule, your palms become sweaty, your knuckles turn white, or you wish you could go home?
- Have you had the experience of complex patients who were easier to manage because of a successful collaboration with a mental health professional, or patients who became difficult because collaboration and communication were absent or impractical?
- Do you have patients with multiple volumes of medical charts who are well known to the clinic receptionist and nurses and who appear to spend more time in the clinic than at home?
- Have you discussed among yourselves what collaboration might look like in the clinic and how and where the mental health professional would work, for example, within the main traffic flow of the clinic or on another floor in the back of the clinic?
- Is there a consensus about specific clinical issues to address or types of patients to refer?
- Have you thought about some of the practical details of having a mental health professional become a part of the primary care team (how to refer, schedule, give feedback)?

If there are positive responses to these questions, then the mental health professional can initiate the evaluation phase by providing the clinic's leaders and the physicians a written summary of their findings. The written summary should include the clinic's goals for an integrated care practice, the specific problems to address, and the proposed next steps for future meetings. These steps would include assigning responsibilities for allocating work space, addressing finance issues, developing an orientation-implementation plan, and targeting any specific clinic issues. The written summary is not a formal contract but rather draft notes of what was learned in the recognition and engagement discussions. The notes are offered with a request that clinic physicians review them for accuracy, questions of understanding, and omissions, to ensure a mutual understanding and to avoid any misunderstandings regarding the development of an integrated and collaborative practice.

If there has been little or no thought concerning the practicality of integrating a new person into the clinic practice, if there is no consensus about what problems to address, and if the leaders or physicians suggest that the behavioral health profession work outside of the normal traffic flow of physicians and patients, then the clinic is most likely not ready for a substantive change in its current practice. However, this is a good time for the mental health professional to give feedback on what he or she is hearing as a consultant. For example, the clinic may have other important priorities, and, as a result, time constraints do not allow for a thorough examination of these issues or a time-consuming project. The door can be left open for working together in the future, with a suggestion that a follow-up meeting occur in six months to reevaluate the possibility of developing a collaborative practice. Usually the clinic's leaders welcome this approach and contact the mental health professional when the clinic is ready to move forward.

Stage 3: Evaluation (Panel and Population-based Thinking)

Primary care clinics are undergoing profound changes to meet their patients', the federal government's, and managed care's demands for increased accountability, better service, good stewardship of costly resources, and evidence-based (guidelines) and population-based (prevention and reducing risk) treatment (Isham, 1997; O'Connor & Pronk, 1998; O'Connor, Rush, & Pronk, 1997; O'Connor, Solberg, & Baird, 1998; Pronk & O'Connor, 1997; Pronk, O'Connor, Isham, & Hawkins, 1997; Pronk, Boyle, & O'Connor, 1998; Pronk, Tan, & O'Connor, 1999). The mental health professional will need to determine the stage at which clinics and physicians are responding to these new challenges, as well as how an integrated primary care–behavioral health practice might fit.

Regardless of the developmental stage, the evaluation can begin by assessing the mix of the clinic's patient demographics. Statistical information about the clinic's current patients can help the clinic to begin thinking about population-based approaches, as well as interventions for individuals. Therefore, it helps to characterize the population in terms of risk factors, utilization patterns, patient distributions according to place in the lifecycle (child, adult, elderly), and presenting problems. This characterization will allow some clinics to benchmark their performance with the prevention and management of certain diseases against guidelines and published norms. In some areas, entire care systems are publicly compared to one another on standard measures of satisfaction, cost, and quality.

Given the widely differing sophistication and variability of data systems available in clinics, the evaluation can start with simple physician estimates of the type and frequency of problems, by age group, that would be best addressed with an integrated practice approach. In our experience, parenting issues (especially around attention-deficit/hyperactivity disorder, school problems, and adolescence) occur frequently and provide fertile ground for the mental health professional to work collaboratively. Family physicians, internists, and specialists frequently mention chronic pain, chronic medical illness, depression and anxiety disorders, and high utilization of clinic services as appropriate clinical targets for integrated care practice.

If more sophisticated clinical information systems are available, proactive lists can identify potential treatment targets such as care planning for high utilizers of medical services; group treatment approaches for patients with depression, anxiety, or chronic illness; proactive management of common, frequently occurring problems such as job stress, parenting adolescents, and coping with menopause; and development of targeted clinic newsletters and other ways to foster self-management approaches for specific illnesses.

In a 1994 survey of 60,000 patients, out of a population of about 300,000 patients who attended four medium and large primary care clinics in Minnesota, we found that 23% of the patients accounted for 53% of the visits, and 2% of the patients accounted for 10% of the visits (Davis & Heinrich, 1994). Also, each clinic had patients who visited the clinic more than 100 times during the year and at least one patient who had 140 visits! The burning question for the clinic then became, what is the profile of these patients? No immediate answer could be given, but the question stimulated interest in understanding high-utilizing patients and how an integrated mental health and primary care practice could be helpful. The data in these clinics later led to a study of such patients by Fischer, Heinrich, Davis, Peek, and Lucas (1998) titled as "over-serviced and underserved"!

In our experience, most primary care practices are still in the early phases of changing from an acute care delivery design to a flexibly diverse delivery system that can accommodate population-based preventive care, as well as management of chronic illness, team care delivery, and complex care planning. During the evaluation phase, the mental health professional can become acquainted with the clinic's approaches to specific problems, such as the treatment of depression and anxiety in primary care, or the management of the psychosocial aspects of coping with diabetes mellitus, to determine where he or she would be a natural fit.

The mental health professional can build on the clinic's interest in developing approaches to these illnesses. Directed discussion by the mental health professional can facilitate the clinic staff's development of integrated systems of care focused on chronic medical and mental health conditions. They key elements of these discussions could include: referral strategies (who, how, and for what), team-based treatment planning methods such as team conferences, development of team-based interventions, patient self-directed and group treatment approaches, as well as systemic evaluation of the systems and treatments that are put in place. These potential treatment opportunities for integrated practice are also opportunities to build an evaluation and measurement mindset that can fit into an ongoing monitoring of a successful collaborative approach.

Stage 4: Management Plan (from Discussion to Implementation)

OPERATIONAL ISSUES
As the consultation process unfolds, the first meetings and discussions are largely clinical. One of the maxims that has guided our work and provided a solid anchor to keep discussions on target is, "Lead with your clinical foot." This is another way of keeping all parties focused on the golden rule of putting patients first. The ultimate goal is to provide excellent *health care delivery* for patients. However, for the integrated care practice to succeed, a clinical perspective needs strong operational and financial support (see Chapter 3 for more details).

As the conversations articulate and identify important targets for integrated care practice and the clinic is ready to move forward, operational areas must be addressed. Office space, scheduling, transcription needs, patient referrals, messages, mail, medical charts, and progress notes are operational support issues that can lead to or away from the achievement of a clinically and financially sound integrated care practice. When operational issues are not addressed in the beginning, difficulties are inevitable. Often operational details that are not dealt with in a timely fashion can derail the entire process. We learned through trial and error the importance of creating an implementation team involving the clinic administrative leadership and physician, nursing, and clerical staff, to launch a successful integration effort and deal with the many issues that arise.

The immediate task of the implementation team is to understand for what purpose and how the mental health professional will be integrated into the day-to-day clinic practice. Over time, as the glitches of the new effort are worked out, the members of the implementation team will change and rotate based on the current needs of the clinic.

FINANCIAL ISSUES

Simultaneously, the mental health professional and the clinic's leaders need to review financial options to support an integrated care practice. The financial options depend on the existing organizational relationships among the primary care and behavioral health care providers and the mix of insurers of the population being served. Possible organizational relationships include a staff or group model where the primary care and mental health professionals work for the same medical group; independent practitioners belonging to the same provider network; and independent practitioners in separate practices. The typical payor mix of insurers includes various payment methods, multiple insurance companies, and out-of-pocket reimbursement. The various payment methods include:

- Capitated care where a multispecialty medical group serves a large group of members/patients covered by one insurance company and provides medical and behavioral health care for a prearranged amount of money. The medical group leaders make decisions about the internal distribution of the capitation (usually expressed in a dollar figure per member per month) to primary care and behavioral health care.
- Capitation where the insurance company contracts separately with primary care and behavioral health groups to provide care. In this model the behavioral health care is referred to as carved-out care and is often provided by large managed behavioral health care companies. These companies manage a mixture of owned behavioral health clinics and network of contracted behavioral health providers.
- Indemnity insurance where the insurer that pays for care when the patient receives care at the clinic of his or her choice.

Without going into a complex discussion of the financing possibilities and difficulties, the behavioral health provider and the clinic will have different options depending on their organizational relationships and mix of insurance reimbursement. The financial models for clinicians who are salaried by a multispecialty group, which receives the whole health care dollar (a prearranged amount of money for providing medical and behavioral health care), provide the most flexibility in supporting integrated care practice. The medical group leaders can decide on how and where integrated care placement would be effective in improving care to the population of patients it serves. Even though it appears that financial models would be easier to develop when all clinicians are working under the same roof, in actual practice many such medical groups are reeling from the turbulent changes in managed care, archaic billing systems, and separate and parallel financial systems that deal poorly with innovation and novel arrangements. In our experience discussions of these issues by the top leaders of primary care and behavioral health can lead to financial solutions.

In one setting where two of the authors work, there are evolving options for supporting integrated care practice. Mental health clinicians practicing in integrated care placements are now fully integrated into the clinic operations, including the financing and budgeting process. The revenues they generate accrue to the clinic and the clinic pays for their positions. The key driver for successful integrated practice has been a clinical vision of providing better care. Goodwill on all sides to make it work has been aided by external studies and internal data analysis that suggest that integrated care practice not only is well received by physicians and patients but also saves money and physician time (Cummings, Cummings, & Johnson, 1997; Fischer et al., 1998).

For clinicians who are in the same medical group or for patients who have indemnity insurance, an integrated care practice can be supported through separate billing for services, because many managed care contracts actually involve discounted fees for service rather than true capitation. Here, the issues are personal preferences and arrangements of the clinic in terms of integrating billing services.

A more difficult challenge is presented when there are separate capitations for primary care and behavioral health care and the behavioral health services are separated out. This is especially challenging if a large number of patients in the primary care practice have this type of insurance. Some primary care clinics have been extremely creative in responding to these situations. They have credentialed the behavioral health provider as part of their medical group, allowing them to bill for the mental health professional's services. Once compelling clinical reasons have been established to develop an integrated care practice and the mental health professional and primary care physicians have established rapport, then the financial arrangements can be worked out. In some cases, primary care physicians have decided to pay for the mental health professional themselves, because it helps them and their patients, despite the inability to get the costs reimbursed properly.

Indemnity insurance provides the most flexibility for integrated care practice support, as both primary care and behavioral health clinicians can bill for individual time spent with patients. However, in all situations, the mental health professional, with the help of the clinic business manager or administrator, will need to become savvy about medical insurance requirements for documentation, diagnosis, procedure codes, and service fees. When a primary care physician requests a consultation, the procedure codes and reimbursement rates are significantly different from the codes and rates for traditional behavioral healthcare. Documentation of symptoms, diagnosis, and procedure codes for services provided have to be consistent and coherent, or reimbursement may be denied. For psychiatrists in primary care settings, codes representing office examinations and complexity of cases lead to case ratings and differing reimbursement rates for the services provided.

Financial discussions are often the most difficult discussions to have, especially if the financial arrangements are developed prior to establishment of the clinical basis for developing an integrated clinical practice. However, as mentioned earlier, when everyone leads with a clinical perspective and readiness to change is established, then financial issues can be solved in order to move forward with the project. In the next sections, several issues are raised that also influence the successful development of integrated care practices and may or may not emerge during the ongoing regular maintenance and monitoring meetings.

Stage 5: Maintenance (The End of Getting Started and the First 100 Days)

As the mental health professional completes several meetings with the leaders of a primary care clinic interested in collaborative practice, and there appears to be a readiness to move forward, the implementation group completes its work of providing solutions to the issues of space, charts, schedules, and dictation. At this point the on-site work can begin. The last set of issues to be addressed include creating realistic time frames to accomplish goals, making sure that clinic nurses are included in the design process, and anticipating problems as well as hidden agendas. It is helpful to directly raise the issue of the clinic's expectations in relation to the change process. One way to frame this issue is to ask physicians to contrast the amount of time it takes to implement a new medical technique with the time it takes to build an effective physician-nurse relationship or team. Placing goal achievement within the context of developing relationships (primary care–mental health professional and new care teams) can help clinic leaders develop realistic expectations of what can be accomplished and by when. In our experience, it takes six months to a year to get fully established in a clinic, and to learn how to work with nurses, physicians, reception staff, chart room personnel, patient service representatives, and clinic leaders.

The time frame for meeting goals can be reviewed routinely at regular implementation meetings. This is when the composition of the implementation team changes and takes on a more clinical focus. Including one or two physicians and nurses on the team, in addition to clinic leaders, is critical to a successful sojourn in primary care settings. At these meetings, reviewing what is working well and what needs improvement allows everyone to stay informed of progress and engages everyone in solving problems when they arise. Engaging the nurses is particularly helpful as they have a good sense of both the clinic's and patients' needs. In our experience, it is usually physicians who manage the diseases but nurses and receptionists who manage patient care.

At the implementation meetings, some systematic measures of what is changing and by how much can be developed. Measures of satisfaction, such as verbal responses from patients, physicians, and the mental health professionals are a good place to start. This process can be done quarterly or semiannually. The availability of more sophisticated information systems and chart audits allows the evaluation of specific measures of quality or other goals, for example, improving the care of "overserviced and underserved" patients or improving the primary care clinic's care of depressed patients.

During the initial phase of developing an integrated practice, it is important to hold monthly meetings. These meetings provide a forum to address issues or hidden agendas that have the potential to undermine or derail the development of an effective integrated care practice. Often, the "bottom-of-the-barrel phenomenon" will surface, whereby some physicians attempt to transfer patients that they have had on their caseload for years (e.g., those who are frequently demanding, distressed high utilizers of care) to the mental health professional's caseload. Rather than developing a collaborative approach, this is an attempt to have the mental health professional manage these patients without help from the referring physician. The implementation team needs to review such situations, so that a balanced approach include both the physician and the mental health professional.

Chapter 5

An Expanded Identity and Role for Therapists Entering Medical Clinics

Psychotherapists who begin working in medical teams often remark, "This is different than regular mental health." Indeed, working as a member of a medical team in a medical setting (in contrast to a traditional mental health or social service setting) is and should be different. In this chapter we will explore the differences in these two settings by looking at: (1) the differences in focus and purpose between traditional and integrated mental health; (2) the expansion of the therapist's role—what the therapist is attending to in this new setting; and (3) the expansion of the therapist's identity—who the therapist "is" in this new setting.

Traditional and Integrated Mental Health: A Contrast in Focus and Purpose

Behavioral health expertise is most effective when positioned in a health care system in two ways.

1. *Integrated in the medical team:* to help physicians and clinics keep and take care of their patients; as an integrated member of a medical team for patients with psychosocial factors in their overall health concerns, or for physicians who need help in managing psychosocial aspects themselves.
2. *As a specialty service:* to function as a specialty referral service for patients who acknowledge their need for mental health care; a service available to patients and providers.

Behavioral health integration calls for an expanded role with expanded awareness for therapists. Table 5.1 further develops the contrast between behavioral health care integrated in medical care and behavioral health as a specialty service. The right column shows not a difference but an expansion of the traditional scope and role for therapists. The therapist is entering a wider world within which his or her skills are more broadly applicable than in the typical "mental health as a specialty" model. Although the traditional mental health delivery system has historical roots, the integrated model is a welcome expansion for behavioral health professionals.

It is critical for therapists to clarify for themselves "who they are" upon entering practice in a medical clinic. Despite the welcome opportunity, therapists may feel trepidation as they anticipate becoming a member of a medical community.

Table 5.1 Traditional and Integrated Behavioral Health: A Contrast in Focus and Purpose	
BEHAVIORAL HEALTH AS A SPECIALTY *(Traditional Mental Health)*	**BEHAVIORAL HEALTH INTEGRATED INTO MEDICAL CARE** *(Integrated Mental Health)*
Professional model: behavioral health as a specialty service for referral and consultation	**Professional model:** behavioral health services integrated into medical care (mental health provider as a member of a medical team)
Clinical focus: mental health care	**Clinical focus:** medical and all health care
• Separate mental health problems	• Intertwined medical and mental health problems
• Considered the mental health care plan	• Considered part of the medical care plan
• Care of mental illnesses and conditions such as:	• Psychosocial aspects of care for any illness or complaint, such as:
—major mental illness and chemical dependency	—common depression and anxiety, comorbidity
—diagnosable mental health conditions	—somatic symptoms, psychophysio-logic symptoms
—specialty treatment groups and programs	—rehabilitation, back to work
—hospital, day treatment	—complex cases, "thick charts," "difficult" patients

continued on next page

Table 5.1 (continued)

Clinical focus: mental health care	Clinical focus: medical and all health care
–psychiatric emergency, triage –evaluation for any mental health–related complaint –coordination with medical care, nursing homes, other venues for care	–family distress that complicates medical care –chronic illnesses of all kinds –adjustment to illness, adherence to treatment –evaluation and referral for any mental health–related complaint, even if not appropriate for follow-up care in medical setting –coordination with specialty mental health care, hospital, nursing homes, other care venues
Patient view • Patient sees it as "mental health care" • Patient expects exclusive relationship with little coordination or information sharing • Patient self-refers for mental health care or comes to treatment via a referral	**Patient View** • Patient sees it as "health care" • Patient expects team-based medical coordination and information sharing • Patient can call in for medical and mental health care
Offices and working culture • Mental health clinic space and therapy offices • Mental health chart • Mental health clinic systems and support staff • Culture of traditional mental health clinic and professions	**Offices and working culture** • Medical clinic space and exam rooms • Medical chart or quick access to therapist notes • Medical clinic systems and support staff • Culture of medical clinic and professions
Covered benefits and financing • Care limited to diagnosable and covered mental health conditions, as per patient's mental health insurance coverage • Considered part of mental health costs; another referral specialty	**Covered benefits and financing** • Care of any covered health care condition, regardless of mental health insurance coverage • Considered part of medical costs; a member of the in-house medical team

They may be concerned about fitting in; with being attentive, capable, and credible and with not losing professional identity. Indeed joining a new professional community is a change and it is possible to get lost. Therapists joining a medical community can greatly alleviate these concerns by paying attention to the professional identity they take on, or who they "are," upon entering the practice. The bottom line is that coming in with a narrow identity as a traditional psychotherapist is a big risk in medical settings.

Therapists who have successfully joined medical communities have expanded their professional identity or "who they are," and this has automatically made a

---

Table 5.2
Therapist Identity: "Who I Am" and "What I Pay attention To"
In Traditional and Integrated Mental Health

"WHO I AM" IN TRADITIONAL MENTAL HEALTH	"WHO I AM" IN MENTAL HEALTH INTEGRATED IN MEDICAL CARE
• A psychotherapist (4)	• A health care professional (4)
• A member of a mental health discipline or team of closely related	• A member of a very diverse multidisciplinary team (8, 9)
• disciplines (9)	
• A mental health specialist (2)	• A health care generalist (2)
• A "soloist" (6)	• An "ensemble-ist" (6)
• A provider of care for my patient (10)	• A facilitator of improvement in teamwork and the system of care (8, 10)

"WHAT I PAY ATTENTION TO" IN TRADITIONAL MENTAL HEALTH	"WHAT I PAY ATTENTION TO" IN MENTAL HEALTH INTEGRATED IN MEDICAL CARE
• Specific "schools of therapy" (1)	• Generic elements of "good clinician ship" (7)
• Techniques belonging to your discipline (4)	• Care plans that cross disciplines (4, 5, 6)
• Mental health illnesses and conditions (2)	• Common clinical and self-management challenges that cross many diseases and conditions (3)
• The mental health portion of the care (5, 6, 10)	• The entire multidisciplinary process of care for the patient (6, 10)
• Improving the care for this patient (10)	• Improving the total system of care for all patients (10)

big difference in what these therapists see, count as opportunities, have reason to act on, and how they choose to act. This expansion of professional identity is key to being accepted and expanding their skill set in medical settings. Table 5.2 shows how therapist identity or "who I am and what I pay attention to" needs to expand in medical settings, building on what the therapist already is and does. The numbers in the table point the reader to the following discussions. (Portions of the table are adapted, paraphrased, or expanded from Peek and Heinrich, 1995, 1998, 2000.)

1. "Schools of Therapy" and Similarities between Seasoned Therapists

Mastery or dedication to one particular "school of therapy" is not necessary for behavioral health clinicians to work successfully in medical clinics. One particular theoretical background such as cognitive behavioral, interpersonal, solution-focused, or psychodynamic does not make a clinician better suited for primary care or other medical practice.

Mental health professionals interested in medical work settings must be able to expand their professional identity, role, and job description. The more seasoned a therapist becomes in integrated mental and medical health care, the more he or she learns and identifies with the general responsibilities and skills that are required of professionals of all disciplines and all patients. When prospective employers ask applicants to describe their profession, many reply, "I'm a psychotherapist" or "I'm a family therapist." This response implies identification with a particular discipline or technique instead of identification as a health care professional. The therapist's own specific credentials, skills, and techniques remain important but the clinician identifies more with general clinical capabilities than with a particular "school of therapy" or set of techniques.

2. Specialist and Generalist Mindsets

Clinicians initially may approach the topic of behavioral health integration with a *specialty* mindset. Physicians may say to a prospective mental health clinician, "We need help with certain diseases" or "We want you to provide us with certain referral therapies or techniques." Clinicians with a specialty mindset tend to think in diagnostic categories or about specific theories or techniques. However there is also a strong generalist element to health care that is not disease or technique specific, especially for the mental health professional integrated in medical care.

Health care, especially primary care, concerns taking care of a *person*, with a unique set of characteristics, circumstances, problems, and resources. Especially in primary care, the patient is not viewed as a group of independent disorders for clinicians to divide and conquer. The mission of primary care is to take care of people, across all diseases and conditions, including the psychosocial ones. Many of these problems, diseases, and conditions coexist, are driven by similar risk factors, present similar clinical challenges, and freely interact with each other. All of these need to be understood by the patient, family, and clinicians as a whole. Many complex, day-to-day patient care challenges are thought of as generic care management challenges. The term *care management* implies that clinicians go beyond application of their own techniques to the broader task of helping the entire case go well.

3. Generic Care Management Challenges

Experience teaches the value of developing the generic clinician skills and responsibilities needed in the overall process of patient care, whatever their disease or condition. Therapists in medical settings will routinely encounter generic patterns or challenges that emerge while treating many specific conditions, e.g., headache, chronic pain, diabetes, asthma, industrial injury, gastrointestinal problems, and somatization. Clinicians are most effective when they recognize and master the generic care management challenges that commonly arise regardless of the medical or mental health diagnoses. They must also understand specific issues relative to the organ systems or disease processes involved. In particular, the clinician should become proficient in the specific areas that are outlined in Chapter 6, Box 6.1.

Clinicians recognize these generic challenges but often create projects such as integrated behavioral health with specific diseases or techniques in mind rather than with these generic challenges in mind. The care of specific conditions is neither complete nor efficient without mastery of the more general patterns and difficulties that underlie good care for them all. Behavioral health professionals can greatly benefit their patients, their medical colleagues, and themselves by meeting such general challenges that run through much of their work, regardless of the disease. Much of this clinical repertoire is truly general to all clinicians, suitable for use by any health care professional, not just the behavioral health person.

4. Psychotherapy As a Profession or As a Family of Techniques

Becoming comfortable with the generic care management challenges means becoming comfortable with a professional identity that is anchored in the broader picture. One approach that can help is distinguishing one's profession from one's techniques. For example, psychotherapy can be viewed as a profession, but it also can be viewed as a family of techniques. As behavioral health care has many techniques, such as desensitization, hypnosis, biofeedback, family therapy, and psychological testing, biomedical disciplines also have a list of techniques. Yet isn't a profession more than a set of techniques? We think of a profession as having its exclusive techniques, but also offering general capabilities for taking care of people with complex cases in a complex care system.

Clinicians often see patients with significant mental health, behavioral, or life issues factored into their overall health concerns. It is common for patients to think of their pain as entirely biomedical, even when a purely medical approach has little or nothing left to offer them. These patients are unlikely to seek psychotherapy on their own and are often quite reluctant to accept psychotherapy or mental health referrals. Only when the patient links their mental states to their physical symptoms will they consider a mental health referral.

There exists, however, a common pejorative stereotype that psychotherapists do not engage such patients, describing them as "not good therapy candidates." Therapists may probe for psychological explanations, then become frustrated when patients are only concerned with their physical complaints. In this situation, therapists can help clients consider alternative explanations for the pain they have viewed exclusively as biomedical. This does not necessarily look like psychotherapy to the patients. Even though therapists may use the term therapy loosely for this kind of work, they know that the work is about human relationships and suffering, rather than a particular technique of psychotherapy. This broader identification as a health care professional rather than as an applier of specific techniques serves as the basis for collaboration between medical and mental health care.

5. Distinguishing Care Plans from Techniques

When absorbed in the details of their work with a patient's presenting problem, clinicians often do not consider the whole complex situation. Rather they see a case in terms of their "piece of it." However, sometimes clinicians act as though their focused techniques are the whole plan for the patient. This can lead to oversimplified approaches to complex cases, or to multiple narrow approaches prescribed by multiple providers who are not communicating. Patients often complain about this pattern asking, "Why doesn't the left hand know what the right hand is doing?" or "Why do I have to keep reminding my doctors of my other ailments, conditions, medicines, treatments, or concerns?"

We find it useful to teach clinicians to clearly distinguish between a care plan and a technique. A *care plan* is an agreement between the clinicians, the patient, and the family for the care of a specified problem. It includes diagnoses, contributing factors, names of participants, roles, goals, treatments, structure, timing, and all else needed to determine treatment. *Techniques* are chosen for their combined ability to serve the care plan. For example, the care plan for chronic headaches might involve changes in diet, use of medication, muscle relaxation exercises, and improved understanding, recognition, and control of behavioral and emotional triggers. In addition, techniques such as biofeedback, physical therapy, and psychotherapy might be employed to treat the specifics of the case.

6. From Soloist to Ensemble-ist

Health care has many disciplines such as family practice, pediatrics, internal medicine, psychology, psychiatry, social work, advanced practice nursing, and cardiology but is not identified solely by any one discipline. An effective health care clinic or organization combines the efforts of the multidisciplinary practitioners, which is essentially a collaborative rather than a solo effort.

Each member of the health care profession—physician, social worker, psychiatrist, nurse, psychologist, family therapist—can contribute to the patients' care. They need more than ever to share a common ground of good clinicianship regardless of the particular disciplines or "professional ethnicity." The fundamental tenet of good clinicianship is putting the patient first, with each discipline offering its unique contribution.

We think of our profession in the broadest terms as *health care clinician*. As physicians or behavioral health professionals, our specific profession or discipline is one voice in the chorus of health care providers. Emphasizing this helps to develop the common culture needed for collaboration. Literature on the principles and models for collaboration between mental health and medical practitioners has been building (see, for example, Cummings et al., 1997; Doherty & Baird, 1983, 1986, 1987; Maruish, 2000; McDaniel, Campbell, & Seaburn, 1995; Seaburn, Lorenz, Gunn, Gawinski, & Mauksch, 1996).

7. Elements of Good Clinicianship and the Community of Health Care Clinicians

The literature cited above points to the need for better collaboration and community among all clinicians, noting common difficulties such as clinicians of different disciplines not understanding each other, talking past each other, competing with each other, or missing all that is in common in their disciplines. Unfortunately, common pejorative stereotypes exist between medical and mental health professionals, such as these gathered from workshop participants: "On the one hand, in describing the stereotypic physician, therapists respond with 'cold, insensitive, rigid, controlling, egotistical, reductionistic, obsessive-compulsive, pressed for time, technician, counter dependent, and somatically fixated.' On the other hand, physicians describe the stereotypic mental health professional as 'too cerebral, impractical, touchy-feely, wishy-washy, impotent, neurotic, weird, flaky, not a real doc, and psychosocially fixated' " (McDaniel, Campbell, & Seaburn, 1995, p. 294).

Shared practices, decision-making principles, or elements of "good clinicianship" can unite different clinicians or "professional ethnicities" under one flag, so they don't compete and undercut each other and instead take care of patients and families. Such a broad community of health care clinicians is rooted in basic clinical wisdom and good practice across all the disciplines. These are the "elements of good clinicianship" mentioned earlier.

To facilitate collaboration, clinicians need a set of shared practices that will unite them to form a fundamental community of health care professionals. Such practices give them a common basis for planning casework and speaking to each other, even when they do not know each other personally. Over the years we have heard a great deal of practical wisdom from members of various professions. One promising approach to capturing this wisdom is to put it in the form of mottos. These pithy and portable aphorisms serve as reminders, warnings, or decision-making principles that speak equally to all the disciplines. Examples of mottos that reflect practices of good clinicianship can be found in Box 5.1.

8. The Mental Health Professional: Skills and Citizenship

As reviewed in other chapters, flexibility, openness to new ways of working, enjoying team-based work, consultation and support of the physician-patient relationship, rather than individual and separate ownership of patients, are critical to the ongoing success of an integrated care practice.

Box 5.1
Mottos for Good Clinicianship

- *Most difficult patients started out merely as complex.* This reminds clinicians that they can create *difficult* patients just by underestimating how *complex* they are.

- *The right kind of time at the beginning of a case saves time over the life of the case.* This reminds people that it is in everyone's best interest to take time to read all the charts and develop a good care plan, even if "there's no time." Care is better, safer, and more efficient when this motto is followed by clinicians of all disciplines.

- *Patients, providers, and families can't do their part in care plans that they don't understand and embrace.* As a corollary, patient "resistance" is usually a sign of approach, negotiation, or timing problems.

- *Health care relationship problems exacerbate health problems.* This warns clinicians to assess and address patient and family frustrations and anger with providers and the care system. Don't expect good technical prescriptions to work when care-giving relationships are poor.

- *Watch the team score, not just your own score.* This reminds clinicians that the basic outcome is at the level of the whole case, not just their part of it, and what other clinicians are doing needs also to be in their field of view.

- *Care planning is prior to technique application, and techniques are subordinated to the care plan.* This reminds clinicians to make sure their favorite techniques are really called for by the situation. In addition, you must be able to show how every move you make serves the care plan.

- *Managing the disability is often tougher than managing the disease.*

- *When the normal incidence of inconvenient tasks and extra-mile service makes you clench, examine your practice pattern with someone.*

Entering a medical setting for the first time can be quite unsettling for mental health providers. Many of the hallmarks of mental health settings—total privacy, respect for theory, solitary working environments, and 50-minute hours with 10-minute breaks—get lost in the fast-paced environments of medical settings. Different medical groups can create training and socialization experiences to bring therapists into medical settings. The "case rounds" of one group has served as an excellent bridging experience for several years now (see Appendix E for a description of case rounds).

As the mental health professional learns about the specific needs of a primary care clinic and the opportunities for integrated care practice, he or she will need to conduct a self-assessment regarding the fit of his or her skills to the clinic's needs. It is clear that comfort with evaluating and treating the types of problems mentioned in Chapter 7 are prerequisites. Assuming that the mental health professional has the requisite skills, there are additional issues regarding the roles of the mental health professional. One important example is "clinic citizenship," which goes beyond specific skills and training. It refers to the place of the mental health professional within the clinic community. Clinic citizenship can either facilitate or constrain the professional's ability to utilize his or her skills.

Types of citizenship can be compared to the various roles and behavioral options one has by being a guest in someone's home versus being a full-fledged family member. Guests are limited to specific roles and behaviors when they enter someone's home, generally entering only when invited and leaving after the specific invitation has expired. In contrast, family members have differentiated and wider range of behavioral options and obligations such as being present for meals, doing chores, keeping the rooms clean, and differing access to resources within the home. Depending on the age or family role (mother, father, sister, brother), there are many different activities available to each family member and, similarly, different responsibilities and constraints.

To build on the family analogy a little further, families have a built-in hierarchical structure: parents above children. Medical clinics also have their own hierarchy (physicians above nurses and operations staff) that will affect the mental health professional's citizenship and behavioral options. Given the hierarchical nature of the medical clinic and the medical world, the mental health professional will need to elicit and understand where he or she will fit in in terms of the structure. The expectations of the medical clinic regarding the place of the mental health professional can vary widely, even among clinic physicians. The mental health professional will need to take some time to determine the type of citizenship that is available and how it may vary within the clinic. Given the range of possibilities, questions can be raised in some of the early discussions. For example, do the physicians want or expect a regular but periodic consultant (guest) who comes and goes or a full-fledged citizen in the clinic? Full-fledged citizenship comes with opportunities and obligations such as attending all regular meetings, being part of the daily flow of clinic traffic patterns, fitting a patient into the schedule for an urgent problem, being available for hallway consultations, attending conferences, and being open to helping out distressed members of the clinic.

As the mental health professional assesses the various citizenship possibilities that emerge from such discussions, it may be useful to review Doherty, McDaniel, and Baird's (1996) five-level developmental model of collaboration and citizenship.

Level I: Minimal collaboration
Level II: Collaboration at a distance
Level III: Basic collaboration on-site
Level IV: Close collaboration in partially integrated system
Level V: Close collaboration in fully integrated system

As primary care providers and mental health professionals are working on-site and move from basic collaboration on-site (level III) to close collaboration in a fully integrated clinic system (levels IV and V), they begin to share systems (scheduling and charting), communicate by telephone and electronic mail, schedule face-to-face interactions about patients, and coordinate treatment plans for complex biopsychosocial cases with multiple providers. They can begin to think about how to manage panels of patients together, develop shared treatment plans and programs, and can even proactively reach out to work sites, schools, and other community agencies and resources. The emphasis at higher levels of collaboration is on shared and mutual ways of working together, in a more egalitarian, truly collaborative relationship.

However, more likely than not, mental health professionals will enter a clinic where the physician is the team leader by design, tradition, and ownership. Although more recently trained physicians tend to be less hierarchical, mental health professionals may find themselves in a system where they will not be the formal leader of care plans and care teams. However, more often than not, they will become the informal leader for specific patients and care plans. In our experience, issues around power, control, and hierarchy are best dealt with in a non-confrontational way. Utilizing a consultant perspective and assuming a participant-observer role is recommended. From this stance, mental health professionals treat the physicians as coequal colleagues doing their best to improve quality of care. Over time, as the value of behavioral health professionals is increasingly recognized, the issue of leadership or who is in charge tends to fade into the background.

Another citizenship-related concern is scheduling. As a resource, will the behavioral health professional's schedule be open to all and any patients, and if so, how? Are there high-leverage patients who should be referred initially? Are there specific types of patients who should not be referred or scheduled? Does the clinic want the schedule completely booked or kept flexible for urgent consultations or specific patient care conferences? How do the physicians want to receive information regarding patient visits with the mental health professional—weekly updates at a noon care conference, written notes in the chart, electronic mail, or hallway discussions? How will care conferences for complex patients be scheduled? How will team members work together in keeping each other informed and how will each player's role be understood and leadership be decided?

9. Being a Member of a Discipline versus Being a Member of an Interdisciplinary Team

All clinicians are trained in some discipline and must meet its requirements in order to remain licensed as a member in good standing. Psychotherapists and other health care professionals benefit greatly from affiliating not only with their particular discipline but also with other disciplines to form interdisciplinary patient care teams.

Benefits of interdisciplinary team membership include an understanding of other disciplines' viewpoints and identification of common goals. Without these elements, it is easy to become isolated in a particular profession. Additionally, to be effective team members it is important for clinicians to be competent, disciplined masters of their particular craft. Maintaining membership in their "guild," discipline, or community will keep them sharp, so that they are able to receive feedback on their repertoire, and to face colleagues who will let them know good craft from poor craft.

These same guidelines can be applied to health care organizations that employ health care professionals. Health care organizations need to cultivate interdisciplinary care teams in clinics to take care of patients, including teams with mental health professionals. They also need to nourish what usually are called departments, made up of the members of a discipline, to maintain discipline-specific quality control and keep a good supply of sharp players. Organizations need managers who are responsible for building, mentoring, and maintaining teams, as well as managers whose job is to build, mentor, and maintain the discipline-specific "guilds." Organizations also need leaders to maintain a balance between the resources and influence belonging to both teams and disciplines.

Behavioral health professionals entering medical settings will be joining a new, very diverse team. It may contain family practitioners, internists, pediatricians, nurse practitioners, physician assistants, and medical specialists. This is the ensemble with which the behavioral health professional will be playing, and the success of this ensemble will affect the patient's care directly. At the same time, integrated behavioral health therapists should not neglect their affiliation with members of their own discipline or mental health colleagues. This is especially important for therapists integrated in a medical setting as they are likely to be the only mental health professionals in the entire clinic, unlike the physicians. The ability to quickly obtain consultation from respected members of their own profession is essential, even as they function as part of a diverse ensemble.

Integrated behavioral health clinicians can participate in medical clinic meetings. Clinics should coordinate their scheduled meetings with the schedules of the behavioral health clinicians. Group meetings with clinical purpose and content, to various degrees in various ways, can be held. In an established clinic, professional community development takes place as a normal part of clinician relationships, and some teams build up recognized standards of good clinicianship about how to handle casework (see Appendix E for a description of collaborative group meetings). A functional equivalent of case rounds can develop, with high degrees of interdependency, trust, skillfulness, and mutual accountability in the more established clinic teams (Lucas & Peek, 1997).

10. Providing Care for Individual Patients and Improving the System of Care for All Patients

Behavioral health clinicians entering medical clinics are hired to take care of patients, not to create organizational change or facilitate improvement in the care system they work in. However, we believe improving the system of care should be regarded as a constant background task for behavioral health professionals. Behavioral health integration is a response to the problems of separate and parallel systems of medical and behavioral care, as outlined in the Introduction. In this sense, integrated therapists are a central part of an effort to change the care system. Many therapists entering medical clinics are in the first *large* generation of therapists to do so, and hence are in the first wave of therapists trying to change the system of care. All clinicians are involved not only in taking care of *particular* patients, but involved in improving the system of care for *all* patients. Clinicians cannot say, in effect, "I just work here."

Fortunately, behavioral health professionals can contribute a great deal to medical settings such as "systems thinking," and sensitivity to group processes. Many of these sensibilities are part of original training and can readily be applied to the system of care as well as to the complexities of particular cases. While therapists are seldom hired explicitly to bring about changes to the system of care, they are greatly appreciated by all when they step forward skillfully and begin to do so.

A starting place for therapists is to take steps to reduce the fragmentation of health care for the patients they see, even beyond the integration of behavioral and biomedical care. Care that is fragmented across the many transitions, referrals, or shifts between providers, hospitals, and clinics is a well-recognized source of service, quality, and efficiency problems. Systems-thinking therapists who decide to look at the health care system as a large, complex, interacting system can do a great deal for their patients beyond direct therapy services rendered.

Patient advocacy is another way to look at the clinical and systems improvement opportunities for therapists in medical settings. Therapists can advocate for patients in several ways beyond the confines of the therapy session. Therapists can use their "insider knowledge" of the care system to locate appropriate psychoeducational material on chronic pain, weight management, or other resources that patients might otherwise remain unaware of. In this way, therapists can help patients make the best use of their time and benefit from using care system and community resources. Therapists can also help facilitate effective referral processes and make sure the patient receives the right care in a timely manner with minimal fragmentation. Therapists can also ensure that important information about the patient and the patient's progress is understood by the patient's physicians. For example, sometimes the patient sees their therapist on a weekly basis, but only visits their physician every two months or more. If a patient begins to complain to the therapist about a medication side-effect, the therapist might relay this information to the physician or help the patient schedule an immediate appointment. The therapist can accompany the patient to the receptionist and leave a message for the physician. Therapists can talk to family members about the patient's illness, its potential impact on the family, and what the family can do to help the patient or the caregivers. Therapists can visit patients in the hospital, nursing home, hospice, or other care center to maintain continuity of care or psychosocial support to the patient and family. When appropriate, therapists can collaborate with patients or physicians to clarify to insurers what is being done, why, and on what basis the treatment should be paid for.

These responsibilities are often outside the scope of traditional mental health practice; however, accepting them can make therapists' work more rewarding. Therapists in medical settings have the broad opportunity to act as clinicians, patient advocates, and care system designers, which is an exciting opportunity for anyone interested in patients and health care. Even beyond their role as responsible clinicians in evolving organizations, therapists can act as concerned and responsible public citizens in helping improve the societal or policy environment for improved health care delivery through public dialogue and scholarly and professional organizations.

We challenge behavioral health professionals to look at system and organizational factors as part of their work. This may require therapists to emerge from the order and quiet of the professional consulting room to become agents of change. This expansion of professional identity and role to include the care system and changing it is key to the successful integration of traditional behavioral care into medical care at this early stage in its development.

Chapter 6

Ways of Working in Medical Clinics: What Works, What Doesn't

Each year seasoned therapists and new therapist interns are hired to work in integrated, collaborative care clinics. Since an integrated medical clinic is a desirable training site, impressive graduates can be selected to work alongside therapists who have several years of experience working in primary care. The new interns work in a milieu where there is ease, history, and familiarity with collaborative care. However, in spite of these positive predictors of collaborative and interdisciplinary success, there is significant variation from one clinic to another regarding the collaborative care process and how often new therapists are given client referrals.

The Physician Referral: An Important Beginning

Working in a medical setting means that the vast majority of referrals come through physicians or other health care providers instead of directly from patients (Edwards, Patterson, Grauf-Grounds, & Groban, 2001; Reust, Thomlinson, & Lattie, 1999). Many patients in this setting would never darken the door of a mental health office on their own initiative. Their relationship with their primary care physician provides the introduction to mental health treatment.

These patients bring their psychosocial concerns along with their biomedical symptoms to the primary care physician. They seek treatment and assistance regarding these intertwined problems during the 15-minute medical office visit.

Thus, the introduction to mental health treatment via the physician has important implications for predicting the success of integrated mental health care and the individual therapist in a family medical setting (McDaniel et al., 1990, 1992).

To be successful in a medical setting, the typical clinical skills of competent therapists are necessary but not sufficient. Their ability to establish trust, respect, and rapport with referring physicians or other health care providers is equally critical. Therapists who are most skillful in building respectful relationships with physicians are the most successful in obtaining referrals and treating patients.

Qualities of Effective Therapists Components in Collaborative Care

Healthy emotional and interpersonal qualities like self-assurance, openness, efficiency, flexibility, humility, strong verbal skills, and an intuitive capacity to "read" an interpersonal situation are important for therapists to have while working in a medical setting.

Flexibility is a key quality. The typical medical office has a much faster, less solemn atmosphere than a typical therapist's office. Patient visits are scheduled at 15-minute intervals all day long. There is more patient traffic, and physicians are frequently interrupted to take a telephone call or respond to other pressing requests. A medical office has more office staff and patient care (e.g., weight checks, eye examinations, and reading of x-rays) is often conducted in the hallway, perhaps by other nursing staff. In one of our practice settings, the therapy room is located near a pediatric examination room. On several occasions, sessions have been disrupted by the cries of screaming children resisting injections or other medical procedures.

Managed care has introduced challenges that necessitate flexibility. The patient's health benefits, especially mental health benefits, may largely determine the practical range of treatment options. Is the antidepressant on the patient's formulary? Is there a limit on the number of outpatient therapy sessions? How can those sessions be used most effectively? These are questions and potential issues that the medical psychotherapist must consider.

There are no best practices to set up behavioral health professionals' schedules; however, an initial schedule allowing flexibility is recommended so that there is time for consultations and urgent cases. It is also helpful to preempt some of the potential hierarchical problems that often arise during the initial implementation. During the first week or two in the clinic, no patient appointments should be scheduled. Instead, the mental health professional should spend half-days with each physician seeing patients together. This approach will foster mutual collaboration and partnership regarding how to best work together and maximize each other's skills and abilities to provide superior care.

Timeliness and efficiency are also critical abilities. As a general rule, there is a sense of time pressure in a medical office. Since up to 30 visits per physician are scheduled in one day, it is easy for appointments to run over and for physicians to subsequently run behind schedule the remainder of the day. Medical emergencies and patients who need same-day appointments are often squeezed into the physician's full schedule, leading to further delays. The therapist must demonstrate respect and understanding for these time constraints. The mental health therapist should use modes of communication that are the least disruptive to the office schedule. For example, using electronic mail, notes, 5-minute hallway consultations, and other expedient communication methods demonstrates that the therapist understands the time constraints in an office practice. While the mental health therapist might still have some 50-minute sessions, he or she is equally likely to have a 10-minute consultation in an examination room with the patient and physician. Later that day, there might be a 10-minute follow-up phone call with the patient and a quick check-in with the physician to summarize the treatment plan.

Two other qualities are the ability to handle interruptions and the ability to conduct therapy in settings other than a cozy office. On occasion, therapy occurs in the laboratory, the treadmill room, or patient examination rooms. Even if the therapist is fortunate enough to have a designated therapy room, he or she needs to be prepared to work in multiple settings. In addition, the therapist must be able to handle interruptions, such as a physician joining the session midway and staying for only 10 minutes before leaving for the next appointment. The therapist should be sensitive to the needs and expectations of patients in medical clinics, where things are done differently than in traditional mental health settings. The therapist does not need to be apologetic about those differences or try to recreate traditional mental health clinic customs within the medical clinic. Instead the therapist should communicate a willingness to try whatever works.

General Responsibilities for Taking Care of Patients, Regardless of Disease or Condition

Clinicians in medical settings, especially in primary care settings, are asked to assist with a wide variety of patients with a wide variety of diseases or conditions, not just mental health conditions. Generic clinician skills and responsibilities are needed in the overall process of taking care of patients, whatever their disease or condition. Clinicians in medical settings routinely encounter generic challenges resulting from many specific conditions (e.g., chronic pain, diabetes, asthma, industrial injury, gastrointestinal problems, and somatization). Clinicians must understand specific issues relative to the organ systems or disease processes involved *and* recognize and master the generic care management challenges that commonly arise regardless of the medical or mental health diagnoses. Patient care requires more than knowledge of diseases and their treatment, it also requires general knowledge about organizing self and others for effective care and guiding patients successfully through difficult health care experiences. Examples of generic care management challenges are shown in Box 6.1.

Considering the Patient's Needs: A Formula for Successful Collaboration

In an article looking at reasons why physicians are sued, common patient complaints that lead to malpractice claims were discussed. Such complaints include feeling rushed, feeling ignored, receiving inadequate explanations or advice, and spending less time during routine visits. Communication problems and feeling that the physician (or therapist) is indifferent to the patient's needs or feelings is a stronger predictor of malpractice claims than is peer-evaluated quality of care (Levinson, Roter, Mullooly, Dull, & Frankel, 1997).

Levinson and colleagues (1997) noted that many competent health care providers orient patients to the process of the visit. For example, they say, "I will leave time for your questions." This helps patients develop appropriate expectations. In addition, competent health care providers facilitate patient communication by making statements like, "Go on, tell me more about that." They ask patients their opinions. For example, "What do you think caused that to happen?" (Levinson et al., 1997, p. 558). Then, the providers listen to the patients without interrupting. Physicians and therapists can communicate warmth and friendliness by using humor or sharing personal anecdotes, to foster a bond with patients that protects the relationship, even when there is a medically disappointing outcome. Health care providers need to speak the language of their patients, versus using only professional, medical language. And they need to understand patients' perspectives through listening and asking questions regarding the problem.

Depending on their health, illness, and prognosis, patients need varying amounts of support. For example, most primary care offices will have a percent-

Box 6.1
General Responsibilities for Taking Care of Patients,
Regardless of Disease or Condition

- *Managing disability.* Disability is not a disease but a common challenge that is a result of illness or injury. It has to do with helping patients resume life, rather than seeing them gradually become disabled or withdrawn from life. Efficacious care of a disease or injury can still leave a patient with fear, lost connections and momentum, and needlessly diminished participation in meaningful relationships and activities. Helping a person re-engage life realistically but confidently after illness or injury is a common challenge. Sometimes managing the *disability* is a much bigger challenge than managing the *disease.*

- *Ability to coordinate multiple interacting factors and people.* Therapists in a medical setting are likely to see many patients with complex cases, multiple complaints, and inextricable psychosocial and biomedical factors. Their suffering is great and the explanations are not simple. Often many contributing factors, clinicians, social agencies, family members, and treatments and agendas are involved. The chart may be thick or growing rapidly. All this magnifies the importance and the difficulty of patient education, enlisting the patient and family in the care plan, and coordinating all the pieces.

- *Finding the right level of collaboration for each case.* Patient situations vary greatly in their need for collaboration between clinicians, agencies, patients, and families. Cases that involve interacting diagnoses, psychosocial problems, clinicians, and community resources usually require significant collaboration. On the other hand, some patient care situations are straightforward and do not require much of a team to get the job done. The challenge for the clinician is to find the right level of collaboration for each case. Underestimating the need for collaboration means difficulty, delay, poor patient service, and sometimes expensive rework down the road. Overestimating the need for collaboration means needless complexity and expense for both patients and clinicians. Therapists need to know when they need a team and when they don't, by learning to answer the following kinds of questions: How do I know when I need a team and when

continued on next page

Box 6.1 (continued)

I don't? When do I just proceed on my own? When do I make a referral to specialty medical or mental health care that I don't really need to participate in? When do I need consultation to do it right? When do I need to integrate the care in a tight team approach, well orchestrated with a "jointly owned" care plan? When and how do I recognize and address the complex interplay of both biomedical and psychosocial agendas?

• *Maintaining a coherent care plan.* How will multiple clinicians keep track of interacting problems and what they need to do in a given case? Where is the record of the care plan kept? Who will keep it updated? Who will "conduct" the ensemble? How will sudden changes or new information be realistically and rapidly incorporated?

• *Working within a patient's medical conception of the problem.* Therapists often need to treat a patient whose emotional life or mental health symptoms are intertwined with his or her physical complaints and conditions but who insists on a purely physiological explanation and cure. Therapists will encounter patients who do not yet make the connections between physical symptoms and personal realities. Therapists need to learn to "play the ball where it lies" rather than making the patient accept a mental health explanation for the symptoms as a condition for treatment.

• *Understanding problematic health care relationships.* Therapists in medical settings often encounter complex patients whose problems have not responded to previous attempts at care. Sometimes this comes from attempts to treat complex problems as simple ones, poor human dealings, service blunders, or medical mistakes. In any case, skepticism, fear, anger, or great sensitivity may accompany patients to their appointments, regardless of the disease or condition or set of complaints. When confidence and health care relationships are on the skids, technically appropriate care is unlikely to be effective.

• *Understanding family chaos or social poverty that threatens recovery.* It is not uncommon for therapists to find themselves serving patients whose family chaos or social poverty is much more threatening to recovery than the illness itself. For example, patients living

continued on next page

Box 6.1 (continued)

in actively abusive situations or other dangerous social conditions are often swimming upstream when it comes to managing their symptoms and illnesses. Financial problems, social isolation, self-destructive behaviors, resignation, and depressive outlook all can undermine sound medical treatments, particularly when the patients need to participate in their own care (e.g., taking medications, following dietary or other guidelines, and coming to appointments). Often, clinicians find that other services (e.g., educational, vocational, social, spiritual, or correctional) are needed or are already involved.

• *Involving and activating patients realistically in their own care.* Patients and families need to and increasingly *want* to understand what the best care is at any given time, and expect clinicians to negotiate care plans rather than merely give orders. Clinicians need to harness this energy, especially for patients' self-care of chronic conditions. Many patients are already a step ahead of clinicians, having access to much of the scientific information that clinicians have, via health care Internet sites and disease-specific education and support groups, and seeing a great deal of advertising directed specifically at them (e.g., for pharmaceuticals). Clinicians must understand, use, and appropriately customize clinical practice guidelines that are based in research or the best-available practice, and then weave these into patients' own understanding of their maladies. No one clinician can master all the literature and then develop his or her own clinical pathways for every condition, or afford to leave the patient and family outside of the process.

• *Handling difficult patients.* Everyone has had difficult patients or to put it more properly, "difficult patient-clinician relationships" (Keller & Carroll, 1994). This is not just a function of personalities. It is often the clinicians and the care system turning ordinary *complex* cases into *difficult* ones if the complexity is not dealt with well early on— hence, the care management motto, "Most *difficult* patients started out merely as *complex.*" All clinicians need to master the basics of patient-clinician relationships even in complex or trying situations. Such patients are often directed to behavioral health professionals in medical settings, and because of their experience working with relationships and "systems," therapists are in a position to become experts at building or rebuilding patient-clinician relationships in the broad medical context.

age of patients who (1) suffer from chronic illness or chronic pain, (2) suffer from heightened depression and anxiety, and (3) are dying of cancer, heart disease, or some other debilitating illness. These illnesses cause significant pain and distress. At times, these patients are despairing and angry.

Genuine collaboration offers the physician and therapist the opportunity to avoid a defensive posture that subsequently causes them to take the patient's despair or anger personally. Sharing responsibility for the patient means that no one provider need be overwhelmed by the patient's needs. While trying to respond empathetically to the patient's overwhelming life circumstances, providers can still help each other recognize the limits of biomedical science and their own personal limits, and continue to establish appropriate boundaries and expectations.

Hidden Mental Health Concerns

In addition to patients with serious illnesses, health care providers encounter patients with a variety of complex medical and psychosocial circumstances. Many of these patients would never be seen in a typical therapy practice because they would not view their problem as a mental health problem. Therapists need to respond appropriately and sensitively to each circumstance without forcing the patient to accept a mental health explanation for their problems.

Frequently, these patients are equally ambivalent about seeing a therapist in the physician's office. Thus, in addition to treating patients with common mental health problems, such as depression and anxiety disorder, the therapist in the medical setting may see patients who have a more unusual *DSM-IV-TR* diagnosable condition such as somatization disorder, factitious disorder, malingering, and conversion disorder, or no diagnosable disorder at all. A *DSM-IV-TR* diagnosis should not be the indicator of whether or not the therapist makes a particular intervention. While it can be helpful to understand the patient's symptoms and why they are seeking biomedical treatment, identifying a *DSM-IV-TR* diagnosable disorder in the patient solves little.

In their book entitled *The Body Speaks: Therapeutic Dialogues for Mind-Body Problems*, Griffith and Griffith (1994) discussed unspeakable dilemmas or pain that patients face. In response to overwhelming circumstances, physical symptoms can mask or give voice to psychological distress. These physical symptoms often are treated unsuccessfully with traditional medicine. Griffith and Griffith (1994) suggest that these somatic symptoms can be treated only through a safe, therapeutic clinical relationship. This trusting and validating relationship provides a vehicle of safety that allows patients to tell their stories of fear, shame, and threat in a new language that ultimately frees them.

Many of these patients come to their physicians with psychological distress that does not meet the threshold for a *DSM-IV-TR* diagnosis. Some patients may be experiencing a normal physical or emotional reaction to stress. Although the problem is not classified as a mental disorder, the patients may feel distressed and could often benefit from talking to a mental health therapist. Other scenarios include patients with some biomedical risks such as elevated blood pressure but a larger measure of psychosocial symptoms including anxiety or interpersonal conflict. In these patients, the biomedical factors keep the physicians medically vigilant because they can never be sure when the biomedical variables will develop into a crisis such as myocardial infarction.

Frequently, patients with significant psychosocial problems present to their physicians with physical complaints such as headaches, weakness, and fatigue. These patients may initially want only biomedical treatment (e.g., medication) for their physical symptoms. Patients with multiple, vague complaints and significant psychosocial distress such as loneliness, depression, and isolation can frustrate both the physician and the medical staff. Interventions might be necessary at multiple levels—with the physicians, the patients, and the patients' families. Consultation liaison psychiatry specializes in this type of intervention. However, a consultative liaison psychiatrist visits briefly to consult on a particular problem, while the in-house therapist has an ongoing, daily relationship with the medical staff, which can be the foundation for treatment interventions.

At the other extreme are patients who have coped with many challenges and functioned well all their lives but who find themselves unable to cope for the first time when confronted with serious medical illness and the concomitant feelings of overwhelming fear, loss, and confusion. These patients have often prided themselves on their ability to cope with any challenge. A man who tells his physician that he is having a "little problem" facing the fact that their wife of 40 years is dying of ovarian cancer while his Parkinson's disease worsens may be acceptable—it is not incongruent with his sense of mastery and competence. However, a referral to a psychiatrist or a mental health consultant for depression may be outside these patients' realm of comfort.

Most patients fit somewhere between these extremes, and the therapist needs to adapt his or her responses to the unique situation. Conducting therapy in a medical setting is not a "one-size-fits-all" enterprise. In the following sections, we make suggestions that can be tailored to specific clinical situations that arise while working with physicians and their patients.

Recommendations for Therapists

1. Seek common ground or meaning between the physician, the patient, and yourself.
Much research has examined the discrepancies between patient and physician
belief systems (Wright, Kern, Kolodner, Howard, & Branccti, 1998). In some of
these studies, each patient was interviewed shortly after having a conversation
with the physician. During the conversation, the physician gave a brief explanation of the etiology, course, and prognosis for the patient's illness. Often, there
were substantive differences in what the physician thought he or she had communicated and what the patient actually heard. Patients and their families can
create their own meanings and beliefs about illness instead of asking questions.
These beliefs may be based on an Internet chat room, advice from friends or
neighbors, or previous experiences with related problems.

For example, a 69-year-old man who had been a teacher was referred to a
mental health therapist. He was dying of prostate cancer and statistically had less
than two years to live. He was seeking every possible treatment including a pil-
grimage to visit a religious site. Hoping to alleviate the patient's fears and
anxiety, the physician asked the therapist to help the patient address his terror
about dying.

The patient had not told the physician about the alternative cures he was pursuing in addition to the physician's plan. In the initial meeting with the therapist, it became clear that the patient was offended by the fact that his doctor was
"just giving up." The more the physician had withheld treatments such as
chemotherapy, surgery, and radiation, the more desperately and secretly the
patient sought out alternative cures.

In this particular case, the therapist realized that the patient was not at all
interested in discussing his death. While some therapists might have conceptualized the patient's problem as denial, the patient's therapist chose to view it as
a communication problem and issue of comfort and safety between the physician
and patient. Treatment consisted of facilitating a more honest discussion
between the patient and physician.

2. Align with the patients' strengths, including their reason for not needing therapy.
If patients do not leap to the need for psychological therapy, it is important to
avoid talking them into it and to help them explore other coping strategies. For
many patients, seeing a therapist to talk about feelings and experiences will not
be acceptable if their words are reflected back in terms of mental health problems. Align with the patients' strengths and eagerness to cope constructively.
Therapists must adapt to the patient's world view and experience of living and

coping, rather than trying to switch the patient's personal view into a mental health or psychopathology world view.

Depending on cultural background, age, gender, and other variables, each patient has a different perspective on how to cope with problems. Therapy, or talking with a stranger about problems, may not be considered an option. Instead of simply suggesting psychotherapy, the mental health therapist can ask questions to understand the patient's coping skills. Questions the therapist might consider are as follows:

- What has helped you cope with problem X so far?
- Think about some of the most difficult experiences of your life. How did you get through them?
- Many of our patients with problem X have found it helpful to read literature regarding this problem, talk with others with this problem, spend more time with family members, and talk to their priest or religious advisor about this problem. Would any of these be helpful to you?
- What can this office, your physician, or I do to help you face this situation?
- What are you most worried about when you think about Problem X? Is there anything that can be done to ease these fears?

Also, the therapist can point out and compliment the patient on strengths and skills the patient and his or her family have used so far to address the problem. It is humbling to realize that most people have lived their entire lives and faced numerous struggles without ever talking to a therapist.

For example, a primary care physician referred a woman in her early 50s to a mental health therapist because she had been diagnosed recently with chronic biliary cirrhosis of the liver, a gradual degenerative illness with which she would become increasingly incapacitated and finally die. The patient had become increasingly fatigued and eventually needed to quit her job, because she could not work an entire day. Both the loss of an enjoyable job and the diagnosis with its bleak prognosis resulted in symptoms of major depression.

In talking with the patient, the therapist learned that she had worked her entire life, had a self-concept of someone who could surmount any problem, and felt angry about her illness. She was pursuing medical disability and had been referred to the therapist to treat her depression. The patient had never seen a therapist before, nor did she think therapeutic help was necessary.

Noting this patient's pride and sense of mastery (in addition to her hidden fears), the therapist labeled the sessions "coping and educational consultations." The focus of the four meetings was on patient education about what to expect in the future and with regards to achieving personal goals and negotiating treatment in a medical setting. As part of this process, the patient was instructed to conduct an Internet search to learn the most up-to-date information regarding her illness, talk to others with her illness, and note cutting-edge research and issues to discuss further with her physician.

The approach used by the therapist enlisted the patient's strength and supported her self-concept of someone who could deal with problems—even in the face of such an overwhelming illness.

In emphasizing a patient's existing strengths, the therapist can keep in mind suggestions from work on medical crisis intervention (Shapiro & Koocher, 1996).

- Help the patient identify and use social support including family, friends, support groups, the medical staff, and any other resources. Although medical literature is unequivocal about the deleterious effects of social isolation, patients with serious medical illnesses often find themselves alone and frightened.
- Recognize that pain is not pathology and help patients make peace with their losses and dependence. "Patients often lose their original appearance, freedom of movement, freedom from pain, strength, sensory acuity, and ability to communicate or even think clearly. . . . Patients may grieve losses of independence, financial security, occupational identity, family roles, expectations, dreams, hobbies, and even a personal sense of meaning" (Shapiro & Koocher, 1996, p. 111).
- Help the patient know and understand the illness, treatment, and prognosis. In partnership with the physician, at times, the therapist must educate himself or herself about the illness. In addition, help the patient know and understand the medical culture that may include "diseases without cures, incomplete information, long stays in waiting rooms, overworked medical professionals and uncooperative bureaucrats. Patients often need quick survival lessons" (Shapiro & Koocher, 1996, p. 113). Patients must demonstrate competent social skills at a time when they are feeling the most vulnerable, fearful, angry, dependent, and overwhelmed.

3. *Think about treating the patient's social system, not just the patient.* Depending on the patient's social situation, the therapist needs to be open to consultations, telephone calls, conferences, and other forms of communication with the patient's family and friends (assuming the patient gives permission). The therapist is in a unique position to assess for situations where the physician needs to

go beyond the traditional 15-minute office visit and spend time meeting the patient and family to answer questions or to provide information. Therapists can facilitate these meetings (Patterson, Williams, Grounds, & Chamow, 1998).

A compelling argument for treating the patient's entire social system comes from an article in *Science* (House, Landis, & Umberson, 1988). Summarizing data on a multitude of illnesses and death rates among persons with a low quantity and quality of social relationships, these authors concluded that poor and few relationships constitute a risk factor rivaling the effects of health risk factors such as cigarette smoking, high blood pressure, high blood lipid levels, obesity, and lack of physical activity.

4. *Consider the patient's readiness or "ripeness" for intervention.* Unlike patients in a regular psychotherapy practice, medical patients and their physicians expect return visits over a lifetime, as stages of life unfold and episodic illnesses take place. While the model of the family physician treating several generations over decades may be less prevalent today than in the past, physician practices still have far more continuity than those of the traditional psychotherapist. The possibility of seeing patients over time, in sickness and in health, means that interventions do not need to be a one-time experience. The therapist shares the physician's longitudinal approach to care and can establish relationships over time and intervene only when necessary and in ways that are needed.

For example, a physician asked a therapist to join him in a patient interview with a single mother of a 2-year-old boy. The mother was HIV positive. While the actual appointment was a "well child check" (the child was not HIV positive), the conversation turned to the mother's plan regarding caring for the child if she becomes ill or dies. The mother was willing to discuss this briefly as part of the child's visit. However, she declined talking further with the therapist about herself or the child. Over the next year or two, the therapist periodically saw the mother in the office and would usually chat with her casually for a moment in the waiting room or hallway. When the mother's HIV status worsened two years later, she requested meetings with the therapist. These poignant meetings focused on the mother's eventual death and what would happen to the child. It is unlikely that these important discussions would have occurred had the therapist not established trust and rapport before the crisis intensified.

5. *To avoid burnout and to increase new patient access, create therapeutic groups.* Similar to physicians, mental health therapists can quickly become overwhelmed with their patient workload, finding it a challenge to maintain good access for new patients and for return visits. To improve access and reduce burnout, therapists can create therapeutic patient groups for education or support.

These groups can meet in the medical office on an ongoing or time-limited basis. Depending on the patient population, meetings can be specific to an illness or focused on one topic such as pain or chronic disease. While some patients may be reluctant to participate, the therapist can use his or her relationship with the patient as a safe introduction to the group. The therapist can point out the benefits of group treatment such as the ability to build relationships with people who share a given illness. Another benefit is that members can meet outside of group meetings and form a support network. Such groups can be powerful modalities in their own right, in addition to ways for the therapist to save time or improve access and reduce pressure on the schedule.

While some patients may not feel comfortable attending group meetings, groups are particularly helpful in certain situations. Lonely patients with little social support are often pleased to participate in a group. In one clinic, one of us found that isolated, elderly women, many of whom were widows and had children living far away, seemed particularly responsive to group treatments. In addition, patients with an illness for which there is little public understanding of symptoms, such as chronic fatigue syndrome, are often receptive. Patients and family members who face a little-understood, fearsome, and debilitating illness such as fibromyalgia often respond positively to psychoeducational groups that focus on providing information.

6. *Put yourself in the traffic pattern of the clinic, where staff and physicians are constantly running into you.* While many therapists in private practice are used to working independently in a private and solitary setting, this style will not work in a medical clinic. The fast-paced, intense, pressured quality of most medical clinics suggests that the reserved therapist is both "out of sight" and subsequently "out of mind."

In designing the office, some therapists have made the mistake of seeking therapy rooms or offices in an isolated section of the building. The therapist down the hall, on another floor, or in another building may have privacy and solitude but also few patients to take advantage of the setting. Physical space and location either enhance or impede interaction. Therapists should use physical space and time to facilitate the interaction with physicians. For example, keeping the office door open, having an informal consulting office in the hallway, participating in office social events, and being easy to contact are all ways for the therapist to be physically and emotionally present.

7. *Accept interruptions.* In traditional therapy, the uninterrupted session is sacrosanct. In medical settings, interruptions are the norm. Physicians, nurses, and the staff move in and out of the patient examination room, and patients

accommodate these interruptions. Therapists can learn to accept interruptions to sessions and other consultations as part of the ebb and flow of working in a medical setting.

The Unique Nature of Confidentiality

One of the hallmarks of the therapist-patient relationship is confidentiality, an issue that is discussed in detail in chapter 2. In the privacy of the psychotherapist's office, patients are able to discuss secret fears, desires, fantasies, and experiences. They are relieved to learn that what is shared within the confines of psychotherapy is treated with the strictest of confidence, and are often dismayed to learn that there are limitations to confidentiality such as when there is a physical threat to self or others. The preservation of confidentiality is key to patients feeling protected from recrimination or threat in their relationships outside of therapy.

Patient confidentiality, like reimbursement issues, is in a period of rapid change. Patients are increasingly concerned about privacy in general and want greater protection for their medical records (Pear, 1999, 2000). As a way of addressing the public's concerns, some of the following changes could be mandated law in the future (Pear, 2000).

- Information transmitted electronically must be controlled more tightly.
- Health care providers and insurance companies must advise their patients of their rights and tell them how personal medical information might be used or shared.
- Patients must sign forms indicating that they have received information about their rights.
- Only "medically necessary" information can be shared and patients have the right to see their medical records.

These tighter restrictions suggest that prudent medical therapists will want to have an explicit, signed statement from the patient, consenting to a free exchange of patient information between the physician and the therapist.

One way we handle this issue is to provide information about confidentiality as part of the materials given to patients when they see a therapist alone for the first time. Instead of waiting for a specific situation when the therapist and physician need to converse, we address it at the beginning when we are describing our procedures and policies. In addition, we have patients sign a form indicating their awareness of the information exchange. An example of a client-therapist confidentiality agreement that includes the primary care physician is found in Box 6.2. Some large medical systems do not permit extra "home-made" legal-sounding paperwork to be included in the patient's legal medical records. There-fore, the sample form in Box 6.2 is most appropriate in situations where therapist is not working in integrated multispecialty groups that already have specific forms in routine use. Ultimately, it is the therapist's duty to find out what confi-dentiality forms are being used in a particular setting and make sure the appro-priate releases and agreements are in place.

In some outpatient medical practices, both the physician's and the psy-chotherapist's notes (handwritten and dictated) are kept in a separate section in the patient's medical record. In this way, the chronology of medical visits can be kept separate from the chronology of psychotherapy visits, but the medical provider has access to information about the progress of psychotherapy and the psychosocial provider has access to information about the medical treatment. In other medical practices, there is no separation between mental health and medical notes. A therapist working in a medical clinic that is establishing new charting procedures for the first time should think carefully about how to orga-nize the patient records.

Conversations in a medical practice between psychotherapists and physicians are regular and often spontaneous. There is a freedom to share information that may be useful to other practitioners treating the same patients. However, the boundaries of confidentiality are clearly established and limited to the entire treatment team, and patients are fully informed of this practice. Patients are informed that both the physician and the psychotherapist will share information for the purpose of improved care.

Collaborative care is one of the benefits of conducting psychotherapy within the outpatient medical setting (Patterson, Bischoff, & McIntosh-Koontz, 1997). Patients who would not otherwise accept a referral to a psychotherapist are more willing to because of the implicit expectation of coordination between medical and psychosocial care. Skeptical patients are less likely to interpret their physi-cian's referral to a psychotherapist as "there is nothing I can do for you, it's all in your head." More likely, patients can interpret this referral as "I'm still in charge of your care, but there is a psychosocial aspect of your medical condition that needs concurrent treatment." Many patients have expressed comfort in knowing that their physician has unrestricted access to psychotherapy notes and expect their physician to be informed regarding their psychosocial treatment. Patients are relieved that they do not have to tell their whole story to both their physi-

Box 6.2
An Abbreviated Version of a Client-Therapist Agreement

As a client (individual, couple, or family) participating in psychotherapy, you are entitled to information about policies and procedures and about your rights as a client. This agreement is intended to provide you with that information.

Agreement to Treatment

I (or we), _____, give permission for any therapy, testing, and/or diagnostic evaluation seen as helpful by this clinic (name of clinic inserted here) in order to treat me, my marriage, family, and/or other relationships. I understand that therapy may lead to unanticipated emotional stress as well as emotional improvement, and that this clinic does not guarantee any particular results or outcome from the therapy process. I understand that I am free to discontinue therapy at any time.

Confidentiality

I understand that all records, videotapes, and other information concerning therapy will be kept in strict confidence by my therapist. I understand that everything I say to my therapist is considered privileged communication with the following exceptions:

1. I understand that my therapist is required by law and professional ethics to report evidence or suspicion of child, elder, and dependent adult abuse or neglect, with or without my consent.

2. I understand that my therapist is required by law and professional ethics to report threats to physically harm others.

3. I understand that my therapist may break confidentiality by law if there is reasonable suspicion of harm to self.

4. I understand that my therapist is legally obligated to break confidentiality when ordered to testify by a court of law.

In addition, I agree that my therapist may share information with my primary care physician at this clinic in order to coordinate treatment.

cian and psychotherapist. As a result, these patients assume that their physician is just as informed about their family background and other important information as their psychotherapist is. Careful attention to records and confidentiality ensures that patients receive satisfactory health care while clinical information is protected in a way that patients understand.

The Role of the Psychotherapist in Accepting Referrals

In this section we address the scope of practice issues and the role of the therapist in medical settings. To demonstrate the role of a therapist in medical settings, we use difficult patients as examples. Difficult patients are typically those who have exhausted physicians and other providers through noncompliance, playing providers against each another, or overusing services. The therapist's role in accepting these patients is to ease the emotional burden and toll from the other medical providers. Also—and this is where the family systems perspective is particularly helpful—the therapist will help untangle the web of triangulation and recrimination that often exists with these patients. This results in a workable therapeutic relationship between the treatment providers and the patient.

The therapist should have an eye toward how both the patient and the providers have become polarized, and consequently blinded in their abilities to make treatment work. Helping patients and treatment providers communicate with one another, helping patients present material differently to their providers, and helping providers see their patients from a new perspective so they can be more creative in treatment are all within the scope of the practice of the medical psychosocial provider. However, none of these goals is related directly to creating behavioral change in the identified patient, which is the traditional role of psychotherapy.

As a result, the clinician must work outside the traditional role of psychotherapy (i.e., seeing the identified patient as the primary focus of treatment) while working within the medical setting. The clinician should not assume that psychotherapy services is the motivation for referral. If the clinician assumes as much, then he or she will likely fall into the trap (and thus reinforce it) of labeling that has often plagued the referral of difficult patients to psychotherapy, namely, that the referral means there is something mentally wrong with the patient, an "it's all in your head" sort of mentality. Instead, the clinician's job is to listen and to be as creative as possible in tailoring treatment to the specific needs of the physician and patient. As opposed to traditional psychotherapy, treatment may only involve assessment or risk management, and the therapy session may last five minutes or two hours. In each situation, the therapist will coordinate his or her treatment plan with the physician, and will remain in the background unless the physician asks otherwise. The role of the psychosocial provider is much broader than the traditional psychotherapist, but if the expanded definition of treatment is not acknowledged or understood, the clinician will not be as effective or successful.

Psychosocial providers working within outpatient medical settings can keep in mind that the physician making the referral is just as much their client as is the referred patient. It is also important to realize that traditional psychotherapy goals are not always appropriate for patients who are referred within the medical team. Many times, the treatment goal is not to produce behavior or cognitive change in the patient but to aid the physician in bringing about compliance with medical care. For this reason, every referral is appropriate for therapeutic services. It is incumbent upon the therapist to accept referrals as they come, and then find ways of working with patients who do not present as traditional psychotherapy patients.

Also, the psychotherapist should not be surprised by the referral of "impossible cases." This is especially true when the clinic hires its first psychosocial provider. In the beginning, physicians may overwhelm the psychotherapist with their most difficult clients, with whom they have not made much progress or who are not compliant with the medical regimen. Once again, the therapist should not shun these difficult cases, because the therapist is as much, if not more, there for the physician as he or she is for the patient. The psychotherapist must remember that his or her role is to improve patient care within the overall system of the medical clinic and not necessarily to perform miracles by single-handedly producing change in impossible cases.

When we first began working in a primary care clinic, a disproportionate number of referrals from physicians were patients who were noncompliant with medication, personality disordered, excessively demanding, and generally difficult in nature. Physicians were grateful that we readily took on these patients to lessen the emotional toll they were experiencing. The willingness to do so facilitated the establishment of a positive working relationship with the physicians.

Accepting patients, no matter how difficult they may be, is also respectful of the physician's expertise. Psychosocial providers working in medical settings should assume that their physician colleagues are competent in treating many psychosocial complaints. Time constraints, however, inhibit their ability to give these complaints sufficient attention. Referrals are made to psychosocial providers not only because difficult patients have not been making progress in treatment, but also because it helps make treatment more efficient.

Psychosocial providers should clearly keep in mind a biopsychosocial perspective when working with patients. All treatments being provided are interrelated and complementary. Rather than fixing a failed course of therapy, the psychotherapist can address an additional aspect of functioning that aids in treatment. The biopsychosocial perspective is crucial for integrated and collaborative care.

Mind-Body Medicine and the Power of Personal Spirituality

The United States and most industrialized nations have seen a recent resurgence in the use of alternative medicines by patients who are also concurrently seeking traditional medical treatments (Richard, 1998). Results of a 1997 telephone survey of over 2,000 individuals randomly chosen from across the United States revealed a 47.3% increase in the number of visits to practitioners of alternative medicine compared to findings of a similar survey conducted in 1990 (Eisenberg et al., 1998). The authors of this study estimated that Americans made approximately 629 million visits to alternative medicine practitioners in 1997 alone, a figure that exceeds the estimated total number of visits to primary care physicians in the United States during the same year. They also estimated that the out-of-pocket expense for alternative therapies in the United States during 1997 exceeded the out-of-pocket expense for all hospitalizations in the United States during the same period.

More surprising, however, is that almost a third of the individuals receiving traditional medical care also concurrently used alternative medicine therapies for the same condition, and less than 40% of these individuals disclosed the use of these alternative therapies to their medical provider. It is clear from these data that practitioners in outpatient medical settings need to be aware of the use of alternative medicine and need to be open to the reasons behind it.

Awareness of this trend toward the use of unconventional remedies should not be with the purpose of discouraging them. Rather, it should be with the purpose to serve as a more useful resource about these therapies to patients (Fontanarosa & Lundberg, 1998). The more informed the physician and therapist are about the extent to which the patient is using alternative medicines, the more coordinated medical care can be.

Our clinical experience suggests that patients using alternative medicine therapies are more willing to disclose this to the mental health provider than to the physician. When this disclosure takes place, it is not as though patients are trying to tell the therapist to keep this information confidential. It is typically just presented as information about what they are doing to address their physical concerns. The psychotherapist working in a medical clinic is typically in an ideal position to access this information because of their additional time spent with patients.

One of us, when working with a group of women with long-standing chronic pain, was surprised to learn of their attempts to use alternative medicines. The women ranged in age from their mid-20s to their mid-60s and were experiencing pain due to a variety of conditions such as arthritis, peripheral neuropathy, and spinal bifida. The first four meetings of this psychoeducational support group focused on their use of the medical system to address their chronic pain.

During the fifth meeting, one of the younger women casually explained that she had been using herbal medicines and folk remedies to treat her arthritis and that she was currently planning to spend thousands of dollars on an unproven dental surgery that was not covered by her insurance plan. Although she had discussed use of the herbal medicines with her physician, she had not disclosed use of the folk remedies or her plans for dental surgery. This began a discussion of how alternative medicine treatments are received by medical professionals. To the therapist's surprise, all the women in the group had used alternative medicines, including acupuncture, massage, diets, and herbs, to treat their pain. Most of these remedies had not been disclosed to their medical provider. The women were not necessarily afraid of their physicians finding out about use of these treatments but just felt that their physicians were treating their condition medically and that others were treating the condition in alternative ways. Whereas the younger women in the group were more willing both to experiment with alternative medicines and to disclose these attempts to their physicians, the older women were more reluctant.

We are not suggesting that the mental health provider's role is to act as an informant to the physician about alternative medicines the patients are using. To do so would undermine the feeling of trust that is so important to a therapeutic relationship. However, sharing of information to the extent to which it improves the overall patient care and treatment is appropriate; for example, the therapist can help patients become more competent to examine treatment choices and to choose wisely between reasonable and unreasonable therapies.

The Psychotherapist's Role in Discussions of Medication

The mental health provider working in a medical setting does not prescribe medications but must have working knowledge of medications, doses, appropriate usage, and side effects (Edwards et al., 2001; Gitlin, 1990). Knowledge of brain and nervous system physiology is also important so the therapist can understand how medications work to treat various psychiatric and other medical conditions. Knowing the indications and contraindications and the interaction between medications is useful because use of a medication often produces a significant impact on the way in which psychotherapy is provided.

Because of the medical environment in which collaborating therapists find themselves working, discussions of medications become common in therapy. Often, patients will discuss their medical consultations and the medications they are taking. Therefore, knowledge of medications is also necessary in order to coordinate care with the medical provider. It is not uncommon for the medical provider to consult with the therapist about medications, because the therapist is often in the best position to evaluate medication compliance and the presence of side effects.

In our practice settings, patients often discuss aspects of medication usage that are never disclosed to the physician. We speculate that this may be because of the limited amount of time the physician has with patients, or because of the different relationship the therapist has with patients. It may be that patients see their therapist as less of a medical professional and more as a peer and consequently are more likely to disclose information about their medications. Regardless of the reasons, we have consistently found that patients will present information to the therapist rather than the physician. Consequently, the therapist should be prepared to direct some pointed questions about the usage and effects of the medication: Is the patient compliant with the medication? How has the medication affected appetite, sleeping patterns, sexual functioning, and energy level? Are there any side effects that appear troublesome to the patient? Has the patient altered dosage levels because of side effects? Does the patient acknowledge that the medication is relieving symptoms?

Therapists need to be careful in asking these questions so that they do not step outside their realm of professional expertise. They should also be careful not to give advice to the patients about medications. Patients will frequently ask therapists for opinions about the medications they are taking. Often, the best response is to empathetically ask about their concerns and questions and then advise them how to express these concerns and questions (if any) to their physician. Therapists should avoid evasive or nonhelpful responses. It is certainly within the realm of professional expertise of therapists to tell patients what they know about the usage and side effects of medications. However, it is never appropriate to recommend medications to patients, tell patients to alter their dosage or discontinue taking medications, or to suggest that their current prescription is in error. Therapists who believe any of these to be the case should consult with the prescribing physician.

Patients can benefit greatly from the therapist's role as the facilitator of communication with the physician. For example, many of our patients have questions about sexual side effects of certain medications. In this situation, if we know relevant information, we might briefly answer the question. Another option might be to obtain literature including pamphlets and videos from the pharmaceutical companies and let patients read about the medication. Computer-literate patients can do an Internet search. Often these simple steps address the concerns and reinforce the patients' self-efficacy about medication usage.

If more help is needed, the therapist might offer to discuss the issue with the physician or suggest that the patient arrange to talk to the physician about his or her concerns. Prompted by the therapist's discussion of the patient's concerns, the physician might decide to call the patient. In our practice, we sometimes talk to a consulting psychiatrist about the patient's questions and share our findings with the patient. We are happy to serve as a conduit of information in any way necessary to make sure the patient's needs are met.

The Role of Research in Clinical Decision Making

Psychotherapists working collaboratively with physicians must understand evidence-based medicine and the reliance of medical practitioners on research to inform clinical practice. And psychotherapists working in these facilities should be prepared to use an evidence-based approach for their work. Although an argument has been made that evidence-based approaches to clinical work dehumanize treatment, this need not be the case. We agree that a strict reliance on treatment manuals developed for use in clinical trials would be a "cookie cutter" approach to a treatment that is so reliant on the therapeutic relationship for success (Krupnick et al., 1996). Instead, personalizing the treatment protocols in an effort to preserve the therapeutic relationship while at the same time preserving the integrity of the treatment is responsible practice.

But what of the countless psychotherapies that have not been subjected to empirical investigation? Are we suggesting that they not be used? Of course not. However, responsible practice demands that the protocols that have empirical evidence supporting their effectiveness be integrated with whatever approach a clinician is using.

An enlightening series of 33 articles was published in the *Journal of the American Medical Association* (JAMA) from 1993 to 2000 entitled "Users' Guides to the Medical Literature" and subsequently published as books (Guyatt, 1993; Guyatt & Rennie, 2002). Through these articles, readers are walked through all aspects of a medical research report and are instructed in the practical implications of each.

Evidence-based decisions are becoming increasingly important in this age of managed care (Sackett, Rosenberg, Gray, Haynes, & Richardson, 1996). Although the mental health field has not yet been subjected to the same scrutiny as the medical field, third-party payors are increasingly demanding that effectiveness data support treatment decisions (Clancy & Kamerow, 1996). There is not a perfect match between practitioners and third-party payors with regards to the reasons for relying on research to inform practice (Clancy & Kamerow, 1996), but hopefully the goal of both providers and payors is the same: to improve health outcomes (Handley & Stuart, 1994).

Mental health clinicians must understand the evidence-based focus to be able to function in the primary care environment. It answers many questions. For example, it may explain why some physicians do not encourage alternative medicines. Although there are many possible reasons for this, one may have to do with the evidence-based approach to medicine promoted in the field.

Demonstrations of Collaborative Care: Encouragement for New Initiatives

Mental health therapists and their medical colleagues must continue to challenge the status quo and search for innovative collaborative treatment methods that provide holistic care to patients, despite the current era of pressing time constraints and cost-cutting measures (Bray & Rogers, 1997; Burns, 1994). While such innovations are key to a successful future in health care, there is the risk that ideas that may be inconvenient to the typical way of doing things will be neglected due to immediate near-term financial concerns and fear of what is not fully proven. In the words of Don Ransom (1997), "My fear is that giving proper attention to the complex questions of mental health care in the primary context will not seem worth the effort . . . what with so many other pressing concerns impinging on them from this rapidly changing and demanding (medical) environment" (p. 35).

Many of the suggestions in the preceding paragraphs require some changes, energy, and perhaps initial discomfort on the part of therapists and physicians. We end this chapter with a brief summary of the literature demonstrating the success and lessons learned of these initiatives so far. Hopefully, the lessons already learned will encourage fledgling collaborative groups to develop their own style of integration.

In Seattle, at the Group Health Cooperative of Puget Sound, Katon and colleagues (1995) have had considerable success treating depressed patients with a collaborative model that included increased intensity of physician and therapist visits, ongoing surveillance of adherence to medication, and patient education. Results indicated that patients were more satisfied with their care and that patients with major (but not minor) depression improved more than did patients with "usual care."

Another study by Katon and colleagues (1992) examined the impact of collaborative care on highly distressed patients. These patients accounted for a large proportion of all health care costs and often suffered from depression and anxiety. The goals of this study were to (1) affect the primary care physician's care of these patients, (2) improve the patient's psychiatric and functional health outcome, and (3) lower these patients' utilization of medical services (Campbell, 1996, p. 141). The collaborative intervention consisted of a 1-hour diagnostic interview with a psychiatrist and an additional 30-minute interview with the psychiatrist and the physician together. Then, the physician and psychiatrist developed a joint treatment plan to address the patient's biopsychosocial needs. A follow-up conference was held one year later. Results showed that patients receiving the intervention did take their medication more frequently but that their health outcome or utilization patterns did not improve. The authors concluded that a more intensive, collaborative, and ongoing intervention is needed for this group.

Two studies looking at patients with somatization disorder (Smith, Monson, & Ray, 1986; Smith, Rost, & Kashner, 1995) examined the effects of a collaborative, biopsychosocial intervention. Interestingly, the intervention was aimed at how the physician interacted with the patient, not at the individual patient. The intervention consisted of treatment recommendations for the primary care physician, including seeing the patient for regularly scheduled appointments; performing limited physical examinations; validating the patient's concerns; and avoiding unnecessary hospitalizations, surgeries, and other tests. Results from the first study indicated that while there was no change in the self-reported health status of the patients, there was a 53% decline in quarterly health care charges in the intervention group. In the second study, the patients reported a significant improvement in physical functioning, and there was a 33% decline in overall health care charges.

Levenson (1992) reviewed studies on collaborative interventions with chronically medically ill patients. One study that he reviewed demonstrated that cancer patients in brief group psychotherapy lived longer and had measurable sustained immunology changes compared to control group patients (Fawzy et al., 1993). In another study, Spiegel and colleagues (1989) demonstrated that patients with metastatic breast cancer who participated in group therapy showed improvements in mood and pain control compared to control groups (Spiegel, 1993). A third study that Levenson reviewed found that cancer patients participating in group therapy had less distress and better active coping skills than did the control group (Fawzy et al., 1993).

Mental health therapists must continue to focus on each patient's needs and unique life circumstances in order to provide a collaborative approach that heals. As Levenson stated, "Because of our enthusiasm for what we do clinically and educationally . . . we must be careful not to lose sight of the primary goals of psychosocial treatment. The primary purpose . . . is to reduce suffering and improve function" (1992, p. 48S).

Chapter 7

Working with Patients Having the Common Mental Health Problems Seen in Primary Care

Because mental illness is frequently comorbid with physical ailments (Narrow, Regier, Rae, Manderscheid, & Locke, 1993), it is common for patients with mental disorders to initially seek treatment with their primary care physician. Although the primary care physician has mental health assessment tools available, these are often insufficient when the disorder is masked by physical ailments.

Collaborating with a mental health professional can provide valuable assistance as well as greatly enhance the primary physician's ability to accurately assess for mental health problems (Patterson et al., 1996). In fact, research has consistently shown that collaboration between the primary care provider and the mental health clinician is a key element in successfully diagnosing and treating patients with mental health disorders (Bernard & Rasmussen, 1999; Blount, 1998; Campbell, 1996; Cummings, 1997). This chapter highlights efforts that have been made to integrate mental health into primary care and outlines the major mental health disorders that primary physicians are most likely to encounter. A description of the physical symptoms that are often comorbid with a particular mental health problem is given, as are recommendations on how the primary care physician and the mental health professional can work together to effectively treat the mental health patient in the primary care setting.

Efforts to Integrate Mental Health into Primary Care

In recent years, several health care provider groups have begun exploring models of integrating mental health into primary care (Patterson et al., 1997). Some of the groups that are leading the way are Group Health Cooperative of Puget Sound in Seattle, Harvard Pilgrim Health Care in Boston, HealthPartners in Minneapolis-St. Paul, and Northern California Kaiser Permanente (Moran, 1999). The efforts made by these health care provider groups challenge the trends toward increasing fragmentation and specialization.

A research review conducted by the North American Primary Care Research Group (NAPCRG) confirmed that a large percentage of patients with mental health problems, especially those with depression, are treated solely by their primary care providers (Klinkman & Okkes, 1998). In response to the data of undiagnosed mental disorders in primary care, the National Institute of Mental Health/Agency for Health Care Policy and Research created the screen-detect-treat-improve clinical paradigm (Klinkman & Okkes, 1998). The results of clinical trials of enhanced detection and treatment protocols largely failed to show improved patient outcomes and in some cases there was no difference in "usual care" and treatment groups (Klinkman & Okkes, 1998). Although it is not clear why these screening initiatives failed to improve patient outcomes, they did identify several concerns that psychosocial providers should consider. Chief among the concerns found by the NAPCRG Task Force on Mental Health is that none of the initiatives in the study considered comorbidity (including multiple mental health problems or mental health and traditional biomedical illnesses, e.g., cancer and depression). The initiatives also failed to consider the efficacy-effectiveness gap, which refers to the fact that many laboratory-created treatments have concomitant tight controls that do not correlate well to the real world setting of the busy primary care physician (Howard, 1986).

Most Frequently Seen Mental Health Problems in the Primary Care Setting

There is a general consensus that the most common mental health problems seen in primary care are depression, anxiety, substance abuse, and eating, sleeping, somatization, and sexual disorders (Ormel, Koeter, Brink, & Williege, 1991).

Additional disorders commonly seen are specific anxiety disorders such as social phobia, panic, and obsessive compulsive disorder. Other problems include family violence, problems associated with children and adolescence such as attention deficit disorders, and chronic pain and its accompanying psychological effects. Occasionally patients with reality distortions such as those indicating a psychotic disorder are also initially seen in primary care.

The frequency of mental health problems in primary care is not surprising when one considers the overall prevalence of mental health disorders in the United States population (Kessler et al., 1994). A national survey found that nearly half of all respondents reported at least one lifetime disorder, and almost 30% reported at least one disorder in the last 12 months. More than half of all disorders occurred in the 14% of the population who had a history of three or more disorders. Mental health morbidity is concentrated in roughly one-sixth of the population that has had three or more mental health disorders.

Unfortunately most of these patients are never treated for mental health problems, including the 14% with multiple disorders. In fact, less than half of the population with mental health problems receive mental health treatment. Outpatient visits, which focus on vague physical complaints, account for one in every seven primary care visits, and it is during these visits that the physician must decipher the etiology and decide on appropriate treatment for the symptoms.

Besides the alarming number of untreated mental disorders within the primary care setting, research has also demonstrated that the risk of a psychiatric disorder increases as the number of vague physical complaints increases. The number of physical symptom complaints is also correlated with the patient's ability to complete daily tasks, how satisfied they are with their lives, and how often they go to the doctor.

In a study looking at common mental disorders across 14 cultures, researchers found that psychopathology was consistently associated with increased disability and that disability was most prominent among patients with major depression, panic disorder, generalized anxiety, and neurasthenia (Ormel et al., 1994). These studies strongly suggested that patients who request frequent medical care or have chronic medical problems are at increased risk for a mental disorder; thus, it is critical that the primary physician assess the patient for mental health disorders.

Patient Willingness to Use Mental Health Referral

While research has identified some of the most commonly seen mental health problems in primary care, these problems will not be addressed unless the patient is receptive to talking about mental health issues and open to exploring treatment options. Patients with somatic symptoms must be willing to change their approach from looking for a biomedical cause for their symptoms to considering the impact of stress, emotions, and interpersonal conflict in their lives. If the patient is reluctant to consider mental health issues, it is the therapist's responsibility to take the patient "as is" and find a mutually acceptable view of the problem.

Little is known about how physician-therapist collaborative teams divide patient care, but recent work has begun to explore the patient's willingness to use a mental health referral made by the primary care physician. Grunebaum (1996) looked for predictors of missed mental health appointments in primary care settings. Patients with mild distress and those reluctant about seeing a therapist were more likely to miss appointments. In addition, the longer they waited to see a therapist, the more likely the patients were to miss the appointment.

Reust and colleagues (1999) in Springfield, Missouri, had slightly different results. Their findings showed that patients who missed mental health appointments reported financial or transportation difficulties. These patients seemed to have multiple stressors in their lives, and one more appointment felt like an additional stressor and not a possible source of relief. Patients who kept the appointments often reported that a family member or friend urged them to go. These patients also were more willing to admit that they had a mental health problem and that they had tried to work on fixing the problem. Another motivation to keep the mental health appointment was to get or maintain psychotropic medications. One interesting finding was that many of the patients who had initially asked for the mental health referral failed to keep the appointment.

Patient Satisfaction

Thus far, our discussion has focused on structural and physician reasons for separating mental and physical health and patients' willingness to consider mental health issues. Equally important are questions concerning patient interest and satisfaction with mental health care in primary care. Patients' receptiveness to mental health concerns is critical for mental health problems to be identified, as well as treated in primary care. In fact, there is little known about how patients respond to primary care–based mental health. One study compared brief psychotherapy with routine general practice care in which depressed and anxious patients took antidepressants and made more frequent office visits. The researchers found that patients receiving psychotherapy were happier with their treatment, even if their symptoms did not improve much more than those of the routine care group (Friedli, King, Lloyd, & Horder, 1997). Other studies showed that regardless of who pays, patients prefer brief therapies, often no more than one to three sessions, and are likely to quit if therapy extends beyond ten sessions (Goode, 1998).

The informed clinician can be alert for patients with underlying psychiatric issues regardless of whether their initial complaints are physical or emotional. Instead of demanding that the patient's complaint fit into a rigid mental or physical category, the provider can focus on becoming a keen observer and listener. As the patient's story unfolds, the clinician has a variety of treatment strategies, which address the interplay between mental and physical health.

Screening Instruments

Screening instruments are available for primary care physicians to diagnose mental disorders. In some cases, screening measures and methods have improved recognition rates of mental disorders; however, they have not necessarily improved treatment success rates. For a thorough review of psychological assessment in primary care, see the *Handbook of Psychological Assessment in Primary Care Settings* (Maruish, 2000).

The PRIME-MD and the SDDS-PC are common screening measures that were created to help physicians screen for mental disorders in a time-efficient manner (Broadhead et al., 1995; Spitzer et al., 1994; Weissman et al., 1995). The BATHE technique, also a rapid assessment tool, uses a psychosocial interview format and can be completed in 15 minutes (Leon et al., 1995). The acronym refers to the following interview components:

B   Background situation
A   Affect of the patient
T   The most Troubling problem of the patient
H   How is the patient Handling the problem
E   Demonstration of Empathy from the physician, including Background

An additional screening measure is the American Psychiatric Association's miniature *DSM-IV-TR*, which was published specifically for primary care providers (McCulloch, Ramesar, & Peterson, 1998; Pingitore & Sansone, 1998). This manual focuses on nine diagnostic algorithms describing some of the most common disorders seen in primary care. The atheoretical model follows the lead taken by the *DSM-IV-TR* (APA, 2000) in presenting a unitary model of psychiatric and physical disorders, as opposed to making an artificial distinction between the realms of organic and functional. In essence, both the *DSM-IV-TR* and the primary care *DSM-IV-TR* manuals are moving closer to a biopsychosocial model and away from a strictly biomedical model.

Although both manuals recognize that mental disorders may be the direct physiological result of substance abuse, medications, or other general medical problems, weaknesses of both manuals include their lack of focus on comorbidity and subthreshold disorders. Both manuals describe distinct clinical syndromes for the purpose of obtaining rigor and specificity, but these descriptions rarely fit the complex, multilayered problems of primary care patients.

In addition to the rapid screening instruments just mentioned, some pharmaceutical companies replicated screening instruments such as the Beck Depression Scale, the Hamilton Depression or Anxiety Scales, and other scales to assess for social phobia and obsessive compulsive disorders. These scales are made readily available to primary care providers along with drug samples to treat the disorders.

Depression in Primary Care

Demographics

According to a major international study by Murray and Lopez (1997), major depression is the fourth leading cause of worldwide disease burden, after lower respiratory infections, diarrhea, and perinatal illnesses. In addition, depression is the most commonly seen mental health problem in primary care.

Major depression occurs in all parts of the world; however, rates vary widely across countries. For example, the annual rate per 100 adults is 1.5 in Taiwan, compared to 19.0 in Beirut, Lebanon. In every country, the rates of depression are higher for women than men, whereas the rates of bipolar disorder are more equal between women and men. In the United States, the female-male ratio for depression is almost 4:1. Besides geographic location and gender, other worldwide predictors of depression are divorce, substance abuse, experiencing a major loss, and being elderly.

Most people who are depressed experience both a loss of energy and insomnia regardless of their cultural background. A cross-national epidemiological study found that major depression varied in rates across countries but showed similar patterns of presentation (Weissman et al., 1996). The same study showed that both rates and presentation for bipolar disorder were the same across cultures.

Costs

Depression is one of the 10 most costly illnesses in the United States. It has been estimated that the annual cost in the United States is about $43 billion. This estimate includes indirect costs of absenteeism, loss of productivity in the workplace, and premature death due to suicide. It also includes costs for the range of depressive disorders: dysthymia, bipolar disorder, and major depression (Finkelstein & Berndt, 1996). Despite the need to treat depression, mental health care is one of the first services to be eliminated or strictly limited in this era of cost-cutting health care initiatives. This reduction in mental health care is unfortunate because depression is usually a recurrent or chronic medical disorder requiring substantial long-term treatment to prevent the massive personal and societal costs of recurrent illness (Glass, 1999).

Costs of untreated depression include both personal costs to patients in terms of functioning and well-being and financial costs incurred by the patient, his or her employer, and society at large. Depressed patients tend to have worse physical, social, and role functioning in addition to poorer health and greater bodily pain than do patients without depression. One study found that the number of days in bed or bodily pain associated with depression was greater than the comparable association with hypertension, diabetes, and arthritis (Wells et al., 1989). The vast majority of the cost of depression to employers is not for treatment but is from absenteeism and lost productivity (Hirschfield et al., 1997). Taking a strictly monetary perspective, it is cost-effective to treat depression because treatment improves overall functioning, including performance in the workplace.

The costs of treating depression are difficult to measure because patients do not usually present themselves as being depressed. Instead they show up at the emergency department complaining of pain, missed days of work, and a failure to complete the tasks of daily living. Since depression is frequently comorbid with other illnesses, the costs of treating the other illnesses often include the hidden costs of treating depression. Costs include both the medical costs of treating depression and indirect costs, which are difficult to measure as they are often overlooked. For example, a patient is depressed and misses work because of fatigue and lack of energy, but the loss of productivity is rarely viewed as an effect of depression.

Unutzer and colleagues (1997) conducted a study that looked at the overall costs of health services in elderly, depressed HMO patients, and summarized their results by stating that depressive symptoms were common, persistent, and associated with a significant increase in the costs of general medical services.

This increase was seen for every component of health care costs and was not accounted for by an increase in specialty mental health care. The increase in health care costs remained significant after adjusting for differences in age, sex, and chronic medical illnesses.

It is common for people with serious depressive symptoms to be undiagnosed and untreated (Coyne, Schwenk, & Fechner-Bates, 1995; Keller, Klerman, et al., 1982; Keller, Lavori, et al., 1986). The patients who are treated are most likely to receive treatment from their primary care physician; therefore, it is important for primary care physicians to recognize the typical problems that coexist with depression. For example, it is common for chronically ill patients, patients facing life-threatening illnesses such as heart disease or cancer, elderly patients with declining health, and patients facing major life changes, such as the death of a spouse, to suffer from depression. Whether or not a coexisting problem is present, there are common symptoms that usually occur with depression.

Recognizing Depression

Depression is characterized by a change in appetite, weight, sleep, and psychomotor activity; decreased energy; feelings of worthlessness or guilt; and difficulty thinking, concentrating, and making decisions. In addition, depressed people often have images of dying and thoughts about suicide. Most people who experience depression encounter their first major depression in their late teens or early 20s.

The specifics of the *DSM-IV-TR* criteria for depressive disorders include major depression, bipolar disorder, dysthymia, and adjustment disorders with depressed mood, and are a good starting point to consider when evaluating a patient for depression; however, these criteria are not sufficient screening devices in primary care. Compared to specialist mental health care, most patients do not come to their physician complaining of depression. Instead, depression is masked in a variety of vague complaints, comorbid with another physical or mental disorder, or subsumed by the more dramatic presentation of substance abuse (Starkstein & Robinson, 1989). Chronic pain and chronically ill patients often receive treatment for multiple problems that include everything but depression treatment and patients that are dying are often overlooked when in comes to identifying and treating depression.

One physician described the process of recognizing depression in one of his favorite patients, a man who loved to bowl. Depression had affected both his work and his sex life, but he didn't go see a psychiatrist until he lost his pleasure in bowling and his score dropped. "Ordinarily, when I get a strike I have a little

'Yeah,' " the patient told him. "But once I became depressed, when I got a strike I wouldn't get my 'Yeah.' " The physician suggested that depression is a disease where the "Yeah" switch in your brain turns off (Schwade, 1999).

Depressed patients may present themselves differently depending on their gender, age, and ethnic background. Depressed women may be withdrawn and barely functioning, whereas depressed men may seem angry and sullen. Depressed children often appear irritable while adults have a more typical presentation of low energy, feelings of guilt, and a self-critical, persistent sad mood. Elderly patients may deny their symptoms when confronted with the suggestion that they are depressed (Blazer, 1993; Caine, Lyness, King, & Connors, 1994). An Asian patient may be reluctant to talk about his or her feelings at all and appear embarrassed or ashamed, while patients from other cultures may feel that it is acceptable to complain about fatigue or lack of interest in sexual activity but may not be comfortable being labeled depressed.

Undertreatment

In spite of its overwhelming frequency and the associated costs, depression often goes unrecognized by medical professionals. When it is recognized, patients are often undertreated or not treated at all. In the National Institute of Mental Health (NIMH) Collaborative Depression Study, only 3% of patients with moderate to severe depression had been treated (Shea et al., 1992). Additional studies showed that over half of patients with a history of depression had never been treated (Dietrich & Eisenberg, 1999; Wells et al., 1989). All of the patients in these studies had moderate to severe depression or long-standing (over 20 years) chronic depression. These findings are particularly sobering when one considers the vast increase in the number of depression awareness campaigns and the availability of medications during the last 10 years.

While recent research suggested that primary care physicians are beginning to recognize depression more frequently, these patients are frequently undertreated. Katon and colleagues (1996) looked at high utilizers of primary care services and found that approximately half were depressed. Most had received no medication or treatment in the previous year, and only 10% had received an adequate dose and duration of medication. In another study, Wells and colleagues (1989) found that only 11% of patients with depression of low severity received medication and 29% of those with depression of high severity received medication. Of patients receiving medication, only 41% received an adequate dose.

There are several reasons why patients suffering from depression are undertreated. One is that many people with depression suffer from subthreshold depression or depression that meets a few of the *DSM-IV-TR* criteria but not enough for diagnosis of a full syndrome. In addition, many depressed people suffer from other physical illnesses, such as myocardial infarction, and the treatment focus is on their physical illness alone (Frasure-Smith, Lesperance, & Talajic, 1993). Substance abusers also are often depressed but treatment is usually confined to their substance problems. Thus, because depression is frequently comorbid with physical problems, it is important for the physician to be able to recognize the symptoms of depression.

The primary care physician's ability to recognize and adequately treat depression is critical, and the presence of a mental health professional can augment chances of recognition and treatment. It is essential to know that patients are often reluctant to seek treatment, especially elderly patients, the group with the highest depression rate. Shame can be a significant barrier to seeking help, as many people still believe that depression is a sign of weakness, something an individual should be able to snap out of, or an indication that the person is crazy.

Identifying the Risk of Suicide

Depressed patients are often at risk for suicide. Most patients who eventually kill themselves tell someone of their plan sometime during the weeks before their actual attempt. It is not unusual for the physician to be the person they tell (Hirschfeld & Russell, 1997). Prior to a suicide attempt, having thoughts of killing oneself is common. In fact, there are 18 suicide attempts for every one suicide and a failed suicide attempt is one predictor of future attempts.

Compared to men, women have higher rates of attempted suicide but lower rates of actually killing themselves. Suicide rates are highest among men who are older than 69 years and among young people. White and Native Americans have higher rates of suicide than do African Americans, Hispanics, or Asians. Seventy-three percent of all suicides in the United States are committed by white men. The most common methods used to commit suicide are using a firearm, poisoning, and hanging.

The strongest predictor of suicide is mental illness, most commonly depression, alcohol abuse, or both. Physicians and therapists should feel comfortable asking depressed patients about suicidal thoughts or plans. Assessing for risk includes looking at sociodemographic factors (age, gender), current life stressors, degree of depression, use of alcohol or other substances, and current thoughts about suicide. It is also important to note that previous suicide attempts or a family history of suicide increase the risk that the patient may attempt suicide (Hirschfeld et al., 1997).

A brief (four-item) screening questionnaire has been designed to identify suicidal ideation in primary care patients (Cooper-Patrick, Crum, & Ford, 1994).
These four questions about (1) sleep disturbance, (2) mood disturbance, (3)
guilt, and (4) hopelessness have successfully identified general medical practice
patients who have a high likelihood for suicidal ideation. In addition to working
with patients identified with a distinct psychiatric disorder, these questions can
be used to screen a general medical population.

Collaborative Treatment

A collaborative treatment model for depression offers the best of both worlds:
medication and talking therapy. While analyses are still being done on whether
medication alone, psychotherapy alone, or a combination treatment works best,
the collaborative team can plan a treatment depending on the individual
patient's needs and preference (Katon et al., 1995; Kocsis et al., 1996; Mynors-
Wallis, Gath, Lloyd-Thomas, & Tomlinson, 1995; Reynolds et al., 1999; Schulberg & Pajer, 1994; Shea et al., 1992).

A panel of depression experts suggests that patient preference should be one
of the most important criteria in choosing a treatment (Schulberg, Katon,
Simon, & Rush, 1999). When the treatment is chosen, there should be regular
patient follow-up and monitoring of treatment adherence, and the mental health
expert should have a prominent role as educator, consultant, and clinician for
patients with severe depression. Research suggests that 40% to 50% of patients
who are prescribed an antidepressant medication will not take it for the
minimum duration that is necessary for treatment (Schulberg et al., 1999); thus,
extended psychotherapy can be critical in helping to prevent recurrence.

Guidelines suggest that the severity of the patient's depression (mild, moderate, or severe) and the sense of urgency for symptom relief can help the physician or therapist make informative initial decisions about treatment (Schulberg
et al., 1998; Schulberg, Katon, Simon, & Rush, 1999). Other considerations
include (Depression Guideline Panel, 1993):

1. patient's health care insurance benefits
2. patient's attitude and beliefs about psychotherapy and medication
3. presence of comorbidity
4. presence of substance abuse
5. presence or absence of social support
6. history of recurring, chronic depression
7. risk of suicide

8. family history
9. knowledge of what has worked for that particular patient in the past

For patients with more severe depression, a combination of antidepressant medication and psychotherapy should be selected as the initial acute intervention, rather than psychotherapy alone. Studies of psychiatric patients with recurrent severe depressions suggests that combined therapy has a significant advantage over psychotherapy alone for patients with severe depression; however, for patients with mild to moderate depression, either choice is acceptable (Schulberg et al., 1999).

Physicians may choose to prescribe traditional antidepressant medication or herbal remedies. Two types of medication that are efficacious treatments for depression are selective serotonin reuptake inhibitors (SSRIs) (e.g., fluoxetine) and tricyclic antidepressants (TCAs) (Simon et al., 1996). However, some research suggested that primary care patients are more likely to discontinue TCAs compared to SSRIs (Schulberg et al., 1999). A treatment that has been used more in Europe but is growing in popularity in the United States is Saint-John's-wort *(Hypericum perforatum)*. While clinical trials are still evaluating its effectiveness, some patients request the herbal treatment for symptoms of depression. Whether it has a placebo effect or not, the patient's belief that the herbal treatment (or any other treatment) could help is an important consideration.

In addition or as an alternative to medication, psychotherapy has been effective in treating depression. Psychotherapies that have been successful include cognitive therapy, behavioral therapy, and interpersonal psychotherapy. Because many family physicians are trained to consider the role of the family system in the patient's life, family-based treatments are also commonly used. Most psychotherapies have similar efficacy rates, and the success of the therapy may have more to do with the therapist-patient relationship, patient motivation, and adherence to treatment recommendations than the theoretical approach used by the therapist.

Effects of Collaborative Care

In a study looking at the effects of collaborative care on patients, Katon and colleagues (1995) showed improved satisfaction with care and more favorable outcome for patients with major but not minor depression when a collaborative model was used, compared to usual care by the primary care physician. The terms "collaboration" and integration" have varying meanings depending on who is applying the ideas. Regardless of the setting, the quality of the physician thera-pist relationship and the opportunity to develop the relationship further are key ingredients. It is assumed that understanding the patient's problems, planning his treatment, and implementing the plan will be done together. An advantage of this model is that more time can be spent addressing problems by combining the physicians' and therapists' time. In addition, each discipline's blind spots can be filled in by the other professional who is looking from a slightly different vantage point. When dealing with difficult patients and discouraging situations, the interaction between group members helps maintain a positive morale for each team member.

Looking at the interchange between mental health and primary care, Little and colleagues (1998) documented numerous communication problems between primary care providers and mental health professionals, specifically when a mental health referral was given. The results of this study highlight the perceived urgency of referral for depressive disorders, the challenge of making mental health appointments, and the relative paucity of communication back to the referring physician.

In summarizing their recommendations for treating depression, the Depres-sion Guideline Panel suggested that future research needs to focus on imple-mentation in daily practice rather than providing more information (Schulberg et al., 1998). It appears that just providing information in the typical primary care office is not always enough to create change in the patient.

Anxiety

Next to depression, the most common mental health problems that primary care physicians and therapists treat are anxiety disorders. About 11% of primary care visits are associated with a chief complaint of anxiety (Katon et al., 1994; Schur-man, 1985). Because many patients worry about their health, concerns about ill-nesses such as heart disease or cancer can easily turn into struggles with the symptoms of anxiety. In addition, many anxiety symptoms manifest themselves physically. While some patients might complain about anxiety, it is more likely that anxious patients will initially talk about physical symptoms or worries.

Costs

Anxiety disorders are costly at many levels, impacting society and the individual from both a financial and a social standpoint. In the United States, people with anxiety use on average twice as many health care services as nonanxious patients (Gauthier, 1997). In addition, families frequently change their plans or lifestyle to accommodate their anxious family member. For example, we knew of a family that loved the outdoors but had to quit camping because of their daughter's terror of spiders. Employment is also commonly affected, as people with anxiety disorders lose productivity in their work setting and patients report that their lives evolve around their disorder.

Quality of life for patients suffering from anxiety disorders can be greatly impaired (Rapaport, 1999). In particular, panic disorder, social phobia, and post-traumatic stress disorder are associated with decreased quality of life. Patients with social phobia may not be able to work or have close relationships, and patients with panic disorder are often on public assistance or disability (Rapaport, 1999). One patient with social phobia reported, "I would be a different person in a different place if I didn't have to deal with this on a daily basis." She recounted a life full of compromises and missed opportunities to accommodate her fears. In addition, anxiety disorders are often accompanied by a host of problems including poor physical and emotional health, alcohol abuse, and frequent thoughts of suicide.

Recognizing Anxiety

Physical symptoms that often indicate problems with anxiety or co-occur with anxiety include chest pain, tachycardia, gastrointestinal symptoms, headaches, faintness, and hypertension. Many patients with anxiety present with somatic symptoms and use medical services frequently, as they make numerous trips to their physician's office seeking reassurance for one symptom or another. Consequently, if these concerns are not addressed adequately in an outpatient setting, these anxious patients are likely to show up at an emergency department, terrified that they are going to die.

Many of the same issues discussed in the depression section also exist for anxiety problems. For example, like depression, anxiety is frequently comorbid with other physical or mental health illnesses, and patients can have subthreshold anxiety such that the physician overlooks the symptoms. For instance, a patient diagnosed with breast cancer may respond to the diagnosis by entering a deep depression. Effective, rapid treatment may eradicate the cancer cells, boost the patient's spirits, and give her hope for the future. However, she also may become increasingly anxious about the chances of recurrence, and each checkup can serve as a reminder of the cancer risk and reinforce her worried, anxious behaviors.

While some patients suffer from anxiety and worries related to every part of their lives, other patients have more specific worries, symptoms, and responses. Identifying the type of worry, symptoms, and patient responses (such as going to the emergency department because of fear of a heart attack or checking multiple times to make sure the stove is off) can help to determine what type of disorder the patient has (Gedenk & Nepps, 1996).

Although anxiety disorders are one of the most commonly seen mental health problems in children, seldom will a family request treatment for a child's anxiety symptoms. Instead, the family will come to the physician because the child or adolescent refuses to go to school, fears some catastrophe is going to befall him or her or the parents, or has few friends because of shy behaviors. Symptoms of anxiety may be revealed in a child or adolescent's fear of spiders, in a compulsive need to count cracks in the sidewalk, or in his or her inability to complete a task.

One explanation for the large numbers of children and adolescents with anxiety struggles is that many anxiety disorders run in families and have a genetic basis. Developmental studies beginning with children suggest that temperamental traits such as shyness and low risk taking are often precursors to anxiety syndromes such as social phobia or panic disorder. In addition, loss or traumatic events during early childhood can lead to lives filled with anxiety. In our clinic, we recently saw a patient who is terrified of dogs because she was bitten by a neighbor's dog when she was a child. Parents brought another adolescent to the clinic because he was failing his speech class. He had good grades in every other subject but refused to give his speeches to classmates and was willing to fail the speech class rather than face public scrutiny. During the interview, it became clear that his source of anxiety stemmed from a past traumatic event, as the boy recounted being humiliated in elementary school when he had forgotten his speech.

Assessment

Some pharmaceutical companies offer rapid screening instruments or have obtained copyright permission to replicate common anxiety instruments such as the Hamilton Anxiety Scale (Hamilton, 1959) or the Beck Anxiety Inventory (Beck, 1990). Other instruments, provided gratis and easy to score, include scales for obsessive compulsive disorder, social phobia, and specific phobias. One of our primary care physicians was talking to a patient about an unrelated physical complaint and noticed the patient counting the lines in the wallpaper. He had an easily accessible, paper-and-pencil questionnaire to assess for obsessive compulsive disorder. Expecting nothing to show up positive (since the physician had been seeing the patient for several years and had heard few anxiety-related complaints), the physician asked her to fill it out. Much to his surprise, the patient had a very high score on the brief scale.

In related work, PRIME-MD questionnaires that were given to patients in primary care waiting rooms revealed several long-term patients who had undisclosed anxiety disorders (Patterson & Bischoff, 1999; Spitzer et al., 1994). This group included patients who had been seeing their personal physician for several years. These patients had failed to mention the extent of their fears and worries, or the physicians had overlooked their comments. Since the clinic where the study was conducted had active mental health professionals working with the physicians, it was striking that numerous patients with mental health concerns were still being missed.

Treatment

Anxiety symptoms can be undertreated or overtreated. For example, a physician might focus exclusively on biomedical symptoms of an illness and ignore the patient's anxiety. A physician also can overtreat anxiety by ordering expensive tests and laboratory work before eventually realizing that fear and worry are the genesis of the patient's complaints. It is easy to understand why medical staff can become exasperated with the anxious, high-utilizing patient and feel that the patient is taking excessive time for what seems to be trivial concerns. At the same time, the patient can feel increasingly desperate as he or she seeks reassurance but finds no relief.

Timing and proximity provide great opportunities for the medical therapist to intervene in these discouraging scenarios. Some anxiety disorders can be treated in a fairly short period of time, for instance, six sessions over a two-month period. Therapists who work closely with the patient's physician can coordinate treatment regimens, patient education, and any medication trials prescribed by the physician.

In our clinic, we have found that the hurried milieu of a busy primary care office causes already anxious patients to become even more entrenched. One of the primary resources the therapist offers is time—time to listen to the patient's concerns, validate the emotional experiences, and suggest alternatives to treating the disorder.

Effective treatment usually falls into three categories: appropriate medications to treat anxiety (and comorbid depression); specific therapies to treat specific fears, usually from a cognitive behavioral orientation; and psychoeducation through tapes, pamphlets, discussion, reading lists, and family meetings. Patients often are open to these treatments when they feel that the therapist and physician understand their distress and are knowledgeable about how to treat it.

Psychosomatic Complaints

The biopsychosocial model that informs this text and serves as a foundation to most collaborative treatment models emphasizes the interconnection between the social, psychological, and physical aspects of a person. As described in the Introduction, the biopsychosocial perspective sees each of these areas as inseparable from the others. Therefore, it follows that physical functioning and health are influenced by intrapersonal or interpersonal stress. Likewise, interpersonal and intrapersonal health is influenced by physical health and functioning. The interdependency between physical functioning and psychosocial functioning is accepted as a truism from this perspective, and therefore it follows that every complaint is psychosomatic.

Most patients with psychological distress have some physiological symptoms, and yet they would not meet the criteria for somatization disorder. Just because a patient has some psychological symptoms (headaches, muscle tension), does not mean he or she has a mental disorder. In fact, somatization disorder is a very strict diagnosis. It requires that there be no physical disorder or the effects of injury, medication, drugs, or alcohol to account for the symptom. If there is a related physical disorder, the complaint or resulting social or occupational impairment is grossly in excess of what would be expected from the physical problem. To be diagnosed with somatization disorder, the person must have 13 somatic symptoms with a duration of at least two years beginning before age 30 (APA, 2000). At the same time, lots of people loosely refer to physical symptoms as "somatization," not necessarily intending the formal diagnosis.

Most of the typical physical symptoms encountered in primary care do have a known physiological pathway (in function, not in disease) and are usually not grossly exaggerated. Actually, when the physician gets to know a patient's whole story, he or she realizes something like, "If this patient wasn't tense and sore given how he is living, then he really *would* be crazy." For example, muscle contraction headaches have to do with chronically tight muscles, often due to being chronically uptight, angry, or fearful. This also applies to other organ systems. The problem is not some kind of lurking mental health disorder called somatization but a set of very tough psychosocial conditions that lead to physiological overarousal and an inability to relax and return to a normal physiological baseline level, usually in one "preferred" reactive organ system. The whole field of "applied psychophysiology and biofeedback" (the name of one organization) pertains to the techniques used to treat these problems, and does not approach them as if they were a mental health disorder called somatization (Hellman, Budd, Borysenko, McClelland, & Benson, 1990).

In one of our clinics, we remember the very human response to emotional pain or stress—responding with physical symptoms—by the motto, "Pain is not pathology." This motto reminds us not to overdiagnose patients who are struggling with multiple concerns or challenges. Often, our clinical responses to patients with physical symptoms indicating distress are no more than common sense. We wonder about the patient's eating, sleeping, exercising habits, and relationships, and look for concrete ways to lessen stress. Often, the experience of talking to a concerned professional is adequate to lessen the patient's symptoms and complaints.

While most psychosomatic ailments can be readily treated, there is a set of psychosomatic complaints that have vexed physicians since the beginning of the profession and for which a special treatment protocol is necessary. Physicians have reported that many of these patients leave them feeling helpless, inadequate, frustrated, and angry. The frustration of working with these patients has been so great for many physicians that some have given these patients pejorative labels such as hateful, obnoxious, and crocks.

What makes these frustrating patients so difficult to work with is that their somatic complaints are often driven by psychosocial stress. Although these patients often have identifiable medical concerns, they also tend to present with conditions that physicians find difficult to diagnose with traditional medical nosology. In addition, these patients do not respond to standardized assessment and treatment protocols (Kashner, Rost, & Cohen, 1995). Consequently, patients who present with variable lists of somatic complaints or undefined complaints are often the ones that no single medical condition or set of conditions can describe.

About a fourth of patients seen in primary care present with somatic complaints that are complicated by or have as their primary underlying causal feature psychosocial distress. Several writers suggested that primary care physicians typically see at least one patient every day that could be diagnosed with somatization disorder (Rasmussen & Avant, 1989). In fact, research showed a prevalence rate of about 5% for somatization in primary care (deGruy, year; Columbia, & Dickinson, 1987), making it one of the most common problems seen in primary care settings.

Recognizing Somatization

Othmer and DeSouza (1985) developed a symptom screening test for somatization disorder that a number of others (Maxmen & Ward, 1995; Rasmussen & Avant, 1999) have advocated for use. The symptoms cover five different bodily systems: respiratory, sexual/reproductive, neurological, gastrointestinal, and musculoskeletal. Othmer and DeSouza suggested that having one symptom pertaining to each of these systems concurrently indicates a strong possibility of the diagnosis of psychosomatic disorder. They argued that because somatization disorder is so prevalent and costly (both in terms of the provider-patient relationship and financially), it is better to treat the condition even if it does not quite meet the full diagnostic criteria. As is true for other conditions described in this chapter, early intervention is typically easier and leads to a better prognosis.

The most common symptoms of this disorder are represented in Othmer and DeSouza's mnemonic, "Somatization disorder besets ladies and vexes physicians." The symptoms identified by this easily remembered mnemonic are: shortness of breath, dysmenorrhea (painful menstruation), burning sex organs, lump in throat, amnesia, vomiting, and pain in the extremities. Othmer and DeSouza suggest that a patient with five of the seven symptoms should be treated for somatization disorder.

Etiology

Because people often experience psychosocial stress through somatic experiences, it is easy to focus on the physiological experience of stress. If the connection between the stress and the physical experience of the stress is not made, the patient will most likely focus on physiological experience, the somatic symptoms, in isolation of the context in which they are present. Consequently, when a patient goes to the physician with somatic complaints and the connection to the psychosocial stress is not immediately made, the somatic experience is reinforced (Lipowski, 1988). Thus, the patient is more likely to focus on the somatic experience of the stress as an indicator of whether something is wrong with him or her.

Besides psychosocial stress, there are a number of other reasons for somatizing. Stuart and Noyes (1999) identified several predisposing reasons such as a history of childhood illness, inadequate parental care, parental illness, and childhood trauma. Other theorists look at current social causes to explain patients' somatizing. Conflict, poor communication, or isolation in the family may serve as the impetus for patients to seek care and attention from their physician.

Somatic complaints then become the ticket into treatment. Acknowledging that psychosocial stress is the cause of the somatic complaints would be admission that a physician is not needed and that perhaps a therapist is. People may be reluctant to see a therapist or to acknowledge psychosocial problems because they do not want to acknowledge that they do not have control over their problems. It is common for people to believe that they can control their thoughts and feelings but that they cannot control illness.

Assessment

Psychosocial stress presenting as somatic problems is often difficult to assess. Physicians attempt to rule out any possible medical conditions that might explain the symptoms. Because many of these symptoms point to legitimate medical conditions for which treatment protocols exist, in many instances the psychosocial root of the symptoms is not discovered until the traditional treatment protocol fails. As mentioned before, the earlier the intervention, the better the prognosis, yet administering a medical treatment exclusively may reinforce the patient's perception that the condition is physiological and not biopsychosocial, which makes a mental health referral later much more difficult.

A variety of paper-and-pencil assessment measures can rule out somatization disorder; however, owing to the widespread prevalence of psychosomatic symptoms that do not meet the diagnostic criteria, the clinical interview is the best source of information. Because of the prevalence of somatization disorder in primary care, we recommend that physicians keep Othmer and DeSouza's mnemonic in mind as they interact with patients, particularly those with whom they are struggling to determine a condition that best represents their symptomatology.

In addition, physicians periodically should ask patients questions about home and family life and work and social interactions to assess for excessive psychosocial stress that may be exacerbating somatic symptoms. Research conducted by Cole-Kelly (1999) suggested that the process of asking questions about family and relationships in the clinical interview does not take much time yet improves patient compliance and satisfaction with treatment, regardless of whether or not the patient has psychosomatic complaints.

Somatic complaints are common for people under unusual amounts of stress. People who are stressed may experience tightness in their muscles, headaches, gastrointestinal problems, chest pains, and a variety of other physical sensations. Also, somatic complaints frequently accompany a number of emotional and psychological disorders. For example, patients with anxiety and mood disorders also frequently report psychosomatic complaints (Rasmussen & Avant, 1989; Slavney & Teitelbaum, 1985). Psychosomatic complaints are also common among patients with psychotic disorders and personality disorders (Rasmussen & Avant, 1989; Slavney & Teitelbaum, 1985) and for couples and families who are experiencing stress within their relationships (e.g., many people get a headache when arguing or lose their appetite or have stomach discomfort because of worry or stress in a relationship).

Treatment for Patients Who Recently Developed Somatic Symptoms

Patients who recently developed somatic problems resulting from acute psychosocial stress and who did not previously consult a physician about these somatic complaints will respond well to empathic reassurance and education. The physician should acknowledge the reality of the patient's somatic experience and explain the relationship between psychosocial stress and physiological experience and illness. The patient can be reassured that as the stress of the situation subsides, so will the somatic symptoms. It is also helpful to provide the patient with advice for reducing stress, in addition to suggesting self-help literature. We recommend that these steps be taken as soon as possible in the treatment process.

If the physician suspects the physical symptomatology is rooted in psychosocial stress, the patient should be given reassurance and should be instructed in stress reduction strategies at the same time that legitimate medical conditions are ruled out. If the physician does this concurrently, the patient most likely will feel that the problem is being taken seriously, which is probably the most important aspect of treatment when dealing with psychosomatic problems. The worst message that the physician can send to a patient is that the pain the patient is experiencing really isn't pain, but is something the patient has made up. This message encourages the patient to prove to himself or herself and to the provider that the pain is real.

Empathic acknowledgment of the patient's problem along with education about somatic disorders is typically something that the physician can do without the participation of the mental health clinician. However, the fact that the mental health clinician works in the same office as the physician can help to facilitate this discussion. Because the primary characteristic of this disorder is an overfocus on somatic experience, it is important that the physician maintain primary control over the treatment being provided. Therefore, the therapist should act as a consultant to the physician. If the physician offers the patient a referral to the behavioral science clinician to help resolve the psychosocial issues contributing to the somatic complaints, and the therapist establishes direct contact with the patient, treatment still should be under the control of the physician, with the primary treatment goal being the reduction of the somatic complaints, not the resolution of the psychosocial stress.

Treatment for Patients with Long-term Somatic Symptoms

When the patient has a large number of somatic complaints that have been present for a long period of time, a different treatment protocol should be used. This is especially true if the patient has had numerous contacts with medical professionals concerning the somatic symptoms. In general, the more failures there have been to help the patient feel better and the more medical professionals that have been involved, the more carefully the collaborative team will need to work together and follow the treatment protocol.

We have found the treatment protocol developed by Rasmussen and Avant (1989) to be useful for somatization disorder. Treatment progresses through three levels. The first level has two goals: The first goal is to develop a relationship in which the patient sees the physician as trustworthy. To achieve this, the physician should patiently listen to the patient's description of the physical complaints and show acceptance of the legitimacy of these complaints. The physician should also communicate to the patient that the symptoms are not expected to abate. The second goal is for the physician and patient to examine the patient's use of medical services and to develop a plan that decreases the number of unscheduled office visits and other patient-initiated contacts with the medical system. Generally it is recommended that patients with somatization disorder be scheduled to see the physician every two to three weeks for a 20- to 30-minute appointment, regardless of the symptom severity. Although some may question the frequency and length of these visits, we have found that the two to three week regularly scheduled visits consume less physician time than the unscheduled contacts initiated by the patient. It also improves patient and physician morale and contributes to the patient's perception that the physician is taking the patient seriously and is trustworthy.

During the second level, the regularly scheduled appointments with the physician continue, but the mental health provider is introduced into the treatment system. The therapist should be introduced as a consultant and as part of the overall treatment team within the medical facility. The patient should be left with the clear understanding that the physician is still in control of the treatment, and that the medical treatment will still be the focus of contact, but that the therapist will help address psychosocial concerns that may be exacerbating the symptoms. It is best if the therapist is introduced within the context of conjoint sessions with the patient until the patient feels comfortable with the therapist and the psychosocial material that is the focus of his or her involvement. The goal at this level is for the patient to begin to gain more insight into the relationship between the physical symptoms he or she is experiencing and psychosocial health.

The goal of the third level of treatment is to begin to create distance between the physician and the patient without leaving the patient with the feeling of being "dumped." The key to success at this stage is for the physician to clearly communicate that the patient's care will continue to be managed by the physician. However, during this stage the patient can begin working with the therapist individually during regularly scheduled office visits, or the therapist and patient can develop their own schedule of appointments that occur with greater frequency than was being done with the physician. At this point, it also may help to begin allowing other physicians or nurse practitioners within the practice to meet with the patient, not so that they can take over treatment but so that the reliance on one physician can begin to be challenged. This will begin to give the patient more responsibility for his or her physical symptoms. In addition, the work of the therapist will help the patient begin to explore the psychosocial dynamic that is contributing to the somatization.

Summary on Somatizing

Respect and reassurance are critical in treating patients with somatization disorder. Physicians and therapists demonstrate their respect by listening carefully to patients' complaints and reflecting an understanding of their concerns. One family physician had developed such a strong alliance with a patient after 10 years of treating him that the patient would now start his doctor's visit by saying, "Now Doctor, I have complaint X . . . or pain Y . . . but I don't know if it is my somatizing problem or not. So I thought I would come see you and we could figure it out." In previous years, this patient had been identified by the office staff as one of the primary crocks of the practice. After demonstrating respect and reassurance over time, the physician established trust so that he could meet his own goals of not ordering expensive and unwarranted tests and procedures. Meanwhile the patient, who needed to feel physically safe and understood, could explicitly ask for what he needed and know he would be treated with dignity. As this example illustrates, once the physician and therapist understand the patient's experiences and concerns, an alliance can be formed with the patient and the resulting treatment is inherently more effective.

Chronic Pain and Chronic Illness

Chronic pain and chronic illness can be the most discouraging experiences that patients and physicians share (Von Korff, Gruman, Schaeffer, Curry, & Wagner, 1997). Both American culture and the biomedical environment place great value in overcoming tremendous odds and achieving victory or, in the case of illness, finding a cure. While other cultures might value being with or accepting pain, Americans are more likely to talk about "beating" their illness. Pain and illness become all-consuming battles, receiving increasingly more time, energy, money, and biomedical resources (Wagner, Austin, & Von Korff, 1996) There is no greater evidence of this battle mentality than the skyrocketing costs of treating elderly Americans with incurable or intractable illnesses.

Recognizing and Understanding Chronic Pain and Illness

Chronic pain usually refers to pain that persists beyond the normal course of healing associated with a medical condition or tissue damage. Chronic pain persists despite the absence of specific tissue damage or a well-defined disease state and is often associated with a progressive disease such as arthritis (Schulz & Masek, 1996). *Chronic illnesses* refer to illnesses that often have no cure, that require lifestyle changes, and that can even change the course or length of a patient's life. Examples include diabetes, cancer, chronic renal disease, and cystic fibrosis.

In our clinic, one of the most helpful metaphors for challenging the win-lose mentality comes from the work of Peter Steinglass. Their chronic illness groups characterized chronic pain or illness as an "out-of-control 2-year-old" (p. 72). In this model, the goal is neither cure nor resignation. Instead the physician, therapist, and patient seek to "find a place for the illness and to keep it in its place" (p. 72). For other views of illness, see McDaniel et al. (1997).

Understanding chronic pain or illness often means knowing the patient's history or experience with the illness. Dimensions of illness to consider include gradual versus sudden onset; progressive, constant, or episodic course; degree of uncertainty associated with the course of the illness; degree of disability or incapacity developing with the illness; and requirements associated with the daily management of the illness (Lazarus, 1985; Rolland, 1984; Schulz & Masek, 1996).

In addition to these variables, we have found it helpful to understand the meaning the patient gives the illness (Wright et al., 1998), the patient's social support, and the patient's hope for the future. In understanding the role of social support, a key predictor of coping, we examine whether the illness is visible or invisible (cerebral palsy versus diabetes). We want to know how the patient has dealt with the chronic problem in the past and assess the level of coping fatigue.

Part of the struggle for many patients with chronic pain is the overresponse or underresponse of the medical system. For example, a patient who usually copes by minimizing problems may resent having to come in weekly for measurements of blood drug levels. A patient with no physiological explanation for the pain may feel humiliated, ashamed, and angry when the busy health care team prematurely reassures her and sends her on her way. To the degree possible, it is important to try to accept patients' explanations of their pain or illness at face value and to actively seek to understand their personal experiences.

An excellent example of coping with chronic illness is found in Christopher Reeve's autobiographical book, Still Me. Reeve, who had been Superman in his acting career, became a quadriplegic from a sporting accident. His book describes his ambivalence about living after his accident until his wife said, "You are still you and I love you." In his book, Reeve describes how his relationships and life became more meaningful after his accident and how he developed a desire to help other quadriplegics by supporting research to find a cure.

Research has shown that patients with chronic pain and illness share core fears and concerns in their lives. Pollin (1995) identified four core fears: fear of becoming isolated, fear of abandonment, fear of being stigmatized, and fear of dying. Pollin also identified four core concerns: losing control over one's life, becoming dependent on others, expressing one's anger, and changes in one's self-image. Schulz and Masek (1996) recommended that health care providers not wait passively for these issues to arise but instead initiate conversations about these issues.

In addition to their pain or illness, many patients have comorbid depression or anxiety (Lipchik, 1998). For example, a patient who is unable to sleep may come to the clinic feeling depressed and in chronic pain. It is often difficult to discern the effects of the depression on the chronic pain or sleep loss and vice versa. If patients have hope and some pleasure in their daily lives, they often can cope better with chronic pain and illness; however, depression and anxiety often rob them of these coping skills. Although a biopsychosocial model reinforces the idea that these are not discrete entities, planning treatments that target each concern usually bring about improvement. Improvement in one area leads to improvement in the other areas. For example, an improvement in a patient's mood will often increase the patient's ability to deal better with chronic pain and to sleep through the night.

Collaborative Treatments

There are numerous traditional treatments for chronic pain or illness (Pollin, 1992, 1994). These treatments include biofeedback, relaxation, finding meaning in one's suffering, pain medications, and behavioral treatments (NIH Technology Assessment Panel, 1996). While each of these treatments work to varying degrees, most patients will be exposed to several of these treatments over the course of their illness.

The NIH Technology Assessment Panel (1996) summarized the findings on behavioral and relaxation treatments by stating that "a number of well defined behavioral and relaxation interventions now exist and are effective in the treatment of chronic pain and insomnia. Relaxation and hypnosis . . . [Alleviate] pain associated with cancer. The evidence was moderate for the effectiveness of cognitive behavioral techniques and biofeedback in relieving chronic pain. Regarding insomnia, behavioral techniques, particularly relaxation and biofeedback produce improvements in some aspects of sleep" (p. 313). While each of the treatments can be given in isolation, a collaborative model that integrates multiple treatment options and is tailored to the patient's specific needs works best. A unique contribution of a collaborative model is that interventions can occur intermittently over time, which is ideal when treating patients with chronic pain or illness. A very important element of the model is the opportunity to bring in the patient's family or other people who are significantly affected by the patient's illness, in addition to giving the patient the opportunity to tell his or her illness narrative (Kleinman, 1988). Although listening is one way to evoke the patient's illness narrative, writing also can be quite helpful. One study examined the impact of asking patients with asthma or rheumatoid arthritis to write about objective measures of disease status (Smyth, Stone, Hurewitz, & Kaell, 1999). The findings suggest that patients with mild to moderately severe asthma or rheumatoid arthritis who wrote about their lives had clinically relevant improvements in health status at four months. Story-telling, writing about one's stressful experiences, and talking with one's family about the pain or illness are all examples of psychosocial interventions that do not require long-term therapy and are ideal to use in a collaborative setting.

Isolated and Difficult Patients

Many patients seen in primary care have no specific *DSM-IV-TR* diagnoses but still have multiple psychosocial concerns affecting their lives and health. These patients often never visit a mental health clinic; however, their psychosocial conditions can powerfully influence their health and their interaction with health care providers.

Social isolation and loneliness are major risk factors for mortality and declining health. A landmark study published in *Science* described increased risk of death among persons with low quantity and low quality of social relationships. Conversely, strong social support can have a buffering effect on health and stress (Spiegel, 1999). While we do not yet understand the pathways between variables like social relationships and health-related quality of life, it is clear that these connections exist. A study by Spiegel (1999) revealed that: "social connection has profound consequences for health. Being well integrated socially reduces all-cause age-adjusted mortality by a factor of 2-fold, about as much as having low vs. high serum cholesterol levels or being a nonsmoker" (p. 1328).

Among the socially isolated patients, there are several types who use the medical clinic as a significant source of social support. These patients include those who are increasingly isolated as a result of their illness and thus come to increasingly depend on the clinic staff for their support, those who have difficulty forming relationships outside the clinic or even with their physician and the medical staff (so-called difficult patients), and those who are struggling with age-related illnesses, such as elderly patients with debilitating health problems.

The first type of patient is the person who has become socially isolated due to an illness. Patients with an illness that causes significant pain, disfigurement, disability, fear, or loss can find that an additional side effect is isolation. This isolation may result from physical or psychological limitations. For example, a diabetic patient who has lost a limb may be reluctant or unable to do much besides go to the physician's office. An illustration of how important the medical office staff can become to a socially isolated patient is revealed in one of our patients who developed Parkinson's disease. This patient's wife reported that many of their social relationships ended because their friends were concerned that Parkinson's was contagious. Since they moved to our community only a year earlier and had no family nearby, both the wife (as the caregiver) and the husband became increasingly dependent on the clinic staff. She brought in cookies and learned most people's names. The staff responded positively to this attention, and when her husband died, she said that the clinic personnel were her family during the difficult period of his illness and death.

The second type of patient is isolated due to poor social skills and may also begin to depend on the medical clinic for social support. Some of these patients may include those with personality disorders (Oldham, 1994). At the clinic, these patients can be dependent and overdemanding, dramatic, self-important and entitled, suspicious, manipulative, or noncompliant. Any of these characteristics can lead to poor social relationships and equally poor relationships with their physician. However, unlike a voluntary social relationship, the physician and staff have to figure out a way to interact with these patients. This process can be challenging and is a great opportunity for collaborative care.

A third group of socially isolated patients who come to depend on the medical clinic are patients whose developmental health needs bring them to the clinic frequently. It seems that both ends of the life cycle—the first year and the end of life—are periods of frequent interaction between patients and medical staff. New parents with infants are frequently anxious about their baby's health and their parenting skills. Elderly patients with multiple health problems visit the clinic more frequently and often look to the medical staff for support.

While we always encourage patients to find support in their everyday setting, we also recognize that some patients need more support from their physician's office, and this is an ideal opportunity for collaborative care. With these patients, the medical therapist can offer time for reassurance, education, listening, and validation of their concerns. This seldom involves weekly office counseling visits. Instead, it is more likely to be brief 10- to 15-minute contacts either during the office visit, over the phone, or by a quick note. Given the profound impact of social isolation on health, the contacts with troubled patients can be viewed as preventive medicine and reflect a genuine interest in patients' lives as well as biological health.

Alcohol and Drug Abuse

Substance abuse and dependence are common problems. However, they are not problems for which people commonly seek medical care. The nature of alcohol and drug dependence is such that the abuser is typically unaware of the extent of the problem until faced with undeniable evidence. This evidence is often in the form of what those in Alcoholics Anonymous call "hitting bottom," which can take the form of losing one's job or family, involvement in a serious or life-threatening accident, or the development of a related, serious physical illness (Alcoholics Anonymous, 1976). Most individuals with substance abuse problems do not identify themselves as such and consequently do not present themselves at their physician's or mental health provider's office for this problem even when intervention is most likely to thwart the most serious of consequences (Washton, 1995).

Unfortunately when a person with a substance abuse problem is seen in the medical setting, the problem is commonly hidden from unsuspecting profession- als during all but the advanced stages of dependence (Washton, 1995). Sub- stance abuse is one of the most frequently missed diagnoses in both primary care and mental health settings. While physicians identify alcohol dependence or abuse in only about half of those patients who should be diagnosed, they are even less likely to identify problem drinking in women (Wallace, 1995) and the elderly (Zimberg, 1995).

With up to 30% of male patients seen in primary care having a substance abuse problem and only half of these being identified correctly, those working in medical settings must become familiar with working with substance abusers. The consequences of a missed diagnosis are severe for the patient, provider, and the medical system in general (Von Korff, 1996).

Recognizing Substance Abuse

Substance abuse is frequently comorbid with, and often a causal agent to, a number of psychiatric and medical conditions. For example, symptoms of depres- sion and anxiety can be produced by the effects of chronic alcohol or drug use on the central nervous system (Beeder & Millman, 1995; Frances & Miller, 1991; Nace & Isbell, 1991). In addition, people who are predisposed to psychiatric con- ditions often use alcohol and drugs as a way to self-medicate for these conditions. Although depression and anxiety may be easier to identify than substance abuse, it is important to treat these conditions while addressing the substance abuse. If these are not treated concurrently, drug use will continue to escalate and only temporary treatment gains will be made (Beeder & Millman, 1995). Besides psy- chiatric conditions, substance abuse also can be either a primary or secondary causal factor in a large number of medical problems. For example, cirrhosis and hypertension are conditions in which substance abuse is implicated. Unfortu- nately, by the time many of these conditions become apparent, substance depen- dence has already advanced to the later stages; thus, it is critical to detect the substance abuse early in order to reduce these deleterious effects.

Assessment Tools

Substance abuse is a problem that can be assessed reliably, rapidly, and easily (Kitchens, 1994) and for which brief intervention is successful when it is detected prior to the development of dependence (Fleming, Barry, Manwell, Johnson, & London, 1997). By far the most widely recognized instrument for assessing alcohol dependence is the CAGE questionnaire (Ewing, 1984; Kitchens, 1994; Mayfield, McLeod, & Hall, 1974). The questionnaire is used in both research and clinical settings because of its ease of administration, its rapid assessment of a complex disorder, and its high reliability and validity. CAGE is a mnemonic for the four questions that make up the instrument: (1) Have you ever felt you ought to *cut down* on your drinking? (2) Have people ever *annoyed* you by criticizing your drinking? (3) Have you ever felt bad or *guilty* about your drinking? (4) Have you ever had a drink first thing in the morning to steady your nerves or get rid of a hangover *(eye opener)*? Advocates of CAGE say that the accuracy of the instrument is improved when the questions are asked as part of a series of questions addressing the patient's lifestyle (e.g., smoking, exercise, diet, and other health behaviors) (Kitchens, 1994).

Other instruments also exist (e.g., Michigan Alcohol Screening Test [MAST]), but their length discourages their use except as part of a pretreatment assessment package (Selzer, 1971). These instruments may be administered more appropriately by a mental health professional once the suspected substance abuser has been referred to one.

As always, the best assessment tool is the clinical interview. Because denial is inherent to the condition, it is important that the clinician approach the patient with an encouraging and optimistic attitude (Liftik, 1995; Miller & Rollnick, 1991; Washton, 1995). We have found that the confrontational approaches encouraged in much of the substance abuse literature have discouraged patients from seeking treatment more than encouraged them. We encourage use of an optimistic approach that focuses on patient strengths and readiness to change (Miller & Rollnick, 1991), and have found this approach to be far more effective at encouraging patient participation in treatment.

Brief Intervention Prior to the Onset of Dependence

By far the best time to intervene in the abuse of substances is before dependence sets in. Intervention at this time is typically far easier, less time-consuming and costly, less frustrating, and more beneficial to health than intervening after dependence has developed. Intervention at this stage typically can occur with minimal effort on the part of clinicians and can be coordinated easily within a collaborative health care team.

In general, problem-focused feedback to patients, goal setting, advice, and professional follow-up result in positive gains during the early stages of substance abuse. For example, one study (Fleming et al., 1997) identified 774 men and women as problem drinkers in 17 primary care clinics. These patients were randomly assigned into one of two treatment groups. In the experimental group, patients participated in two 15-minute interviews with their physician. During the interviews, which were scheduled 1 month apart, the physician provided patients feedback about their drinking and health behaviors, educated them about the adverse health consequences associated with alcohol abuse, and contracted with them to change their drinking behaviors. Each interview was followed up with a telephone call from a nurse two weeks later. Those in the control group were given a health booklet that contained general health information.

A 12-month follow-up found that the experimental group experienced a significantly greater decrease in overall alcohol consumption and number of episodes of binge drinking compared to the control group. These findings were especially true for women. Women in the experimental group reported a 47% decrease in the number of drinks per week after 12 months, while men in the experimental group reported a 44% decrease in the number of drinks per week. The results of this study suggest that relatively brief interventions during the problem-drinking stage can significantly reduce the risk of dependence.

In collaborative care, we suggest that the following intervention strategy be used. After problem substance use has been identified, an interview is scheduled with the patient in which both the physician and mental health clinician attend. During the 10- to 15-minute interview, the patient is introduced to the mental health clinician. The physician provides the patient with the results of the assessment and cautions the patient about the health risks associated with substance abuse. The mental health clinician then can describe the prevalence of substance abuse and provide some education about the psychosocial risks involved. Both the physician and the mental health clinician should then encourage the patient to reduce his or her substance use. The mental health clinician should follow up the interview with a telephone call one to two weeks later. A follow-up visit should be scheduled with the physician and mental health clinician four to six weeks after the first interview. During the follow-up visit, the physician and clinician should assess the patient's substance use, provide additional education, and suggest the option of working with the mental health clinician more closely to establish a plan for reducing the substance use. Self-help literature that the patient can take home should also be available.

Intervention for Substance Dependence

Intervention for substance dependence typically is more involved than for substance abuse prior to dependence and may even include inpatient detoxification. Patients who are dependent often are seen initially by the health care provider because of a medical condition, which may have been caused or exacerbated by the substance dependence. Because of the consequence to physical health, the patient may be willing to change his or her substance abuse; however, some health consequences of the dependence may be irreversible at this point.

The first treatment task is to determine if the patient is in need of supervised detoxification. If this is the case, then both physician and mental health clinician should work together to ensure that the appropriate referrals are made and followed up.

Chapter 8

Working to Promote Healthy Behavior Change (Not Just Treatment of Symptoms)

Preventative Care

Working in a health care system has both opportunities and pitfalls. One opportunity that exists for psychotherapists is to broaden their treatment focus to include preventative care. Historically, most therapists are paid to treat existing mental health problems. Under this system, patients undergo an assessment and are evaluated for a DSM-IV-TR diagnosis or other reimbursable condition. Given that the patient has a diagnosable condition, treatment progresses and is reimbursed according to the condition being treated.

This reimbursement system has reinforced a focus on problems and problem resolution in treatment and has excluded a focus on preventative services. Consequently, even therapist training programs emphasize assessment and treatment of existing conditions rather than stress preventative care. Typically, education on preventative care is not emphasized and is often presented as elective coursework. In practice, preventative care has been relegated to parenting classes and other nonreimbursable services that are paid for entirely by the client. Consequently, most therapists have not included preventative care within their practices. Although this approach to maintaining a practice "pays the bills," we believe that when prevention is ignored, the "whole" patient is often overlooked. This is unfortunate given the potential value of preventative mental health care on long-range physical and mental health. It is also unfortunate given the value of health and health maintenance to many, if not most, approaches to mental health treatment.

Fortunately, modern health care systems stress the importance of preventative care and build preventative care programs into their services delivery packages. While some research suggests that these preventive care programs are often underused, especially by those most in need of them, they provide great opportunities to improve health outcomes (Goldstein, Lobel, Faigeles, & DeCarlo, 1998).

While many therapists bemoan the creation of managed care, one positive result is that psychotherapists can spend part of their salaried time doing preventative work (Patterson and Scherger, 1995). For example, some managed care programs have classes in stress reduction, prenatal health, parenting, cancer education groups, smoking cessation, and lifestyle changes to prevent cardiovascular disease. Many health care systems value therapist participation in these preventative care initiatives. Most health care systems have some preventative care programs in place, although they frequently do not include mental health education. The possibilities for preventative care programs are endless. We know of therapists who offer support groups for caregivers of Alzheimer's patients, and other therapists who teach safe-sex classes to high-risk populations or teach parenting classes to parents of children with disabilities.

The focus of preventative care programs also can be on individuals typically hidden from view but equally in need of support and education. Under the traditional model of providing care, it has been difficult to receive reimbursement for providing education and support to family members and companions of patients with diagnosable conditions. Yet, these often overlooked caregivers and family members experience the stress of the condition, often equally with the patient (Patterson et al., 1998). For example, the wife/caregiver of an elderly patient with Alzheimer's could benefit from patient education, support programs, and other preventative care programs. Preventative care in this instance could help her structure her life and care for herself in such a way that she is not leaving herself vulnerable to physical and mental health problems later. In a traditional problem- and treatment-focused system, the wife's needs and feelings would be overlooked unless she also had a mental health problem or physical condition. Thus, focusing on prevention provides new opportunities for therapists who have historically worked in treatment-based settings.

Broader Focus of Treatment

Working collaboratively in a health care system provides the opportunity for therapists to broaden their treatment scope. For example, in our clinic many depressed patients also have weight problems and many anxious patients have sleeping problems. Psychotherapists historically would have focused on the depression or anxiety alone. Since they were not trained to treat obesity or sleep disorders, they might have overlooked these equally perplexing challenges. At best, sleep or eating problems would be seen as symptoms of the depression or anxiety and these would hopefully be ameliorated as the mental health disorder is treated. Medical therapists working in the health care setting have the chance to focus on issues such as sleeping, eating, exercise, smoking, substance use, stress reduction, social support (developing friendships), as well as specific mental disorders. Indeed, the whole focus of the patient-therapist work may be on preventative skill building.

Today when we see depressed overweight patients, we inquire about their feelings about their weight in addition to assessing for depression. Our depression treatment plan may incorporate a weight reduction component, including having patients weigh themselves before each psychotherapy session. Although asking about weight or sleep is part of the standard of care in the assessment of depression or anxiety, it has now become a common area of inquiry for therapists working in the medical setting. We are able to talk to the providers treating particular "symptoms," coordinate our treatment plan with the treatment that other professionals are providing, and then address or follow the concurrent treatment of weight problems or sleep disorders.

Working with professionals with expertise in many different areas has broadened our perspective when addressing problems. We now ask about a patient's "symptoms" in a different way. They are no longer just symptoms but conditions that have their own legitimate diagnoses and treatments. It is not assumed that if we treat the depression, the person will be able to control her weight or her sleep will improve. Rather, we can now see how these conditions are interrelated (how they affect one another) and how each warrants an individual assessment.

This does not imply that we become the treatment providers for these conditions. If a therapist is not an expert with sleep disorders, working in a medical environment does not automatically make him or her an expert. However, the treatment that the therapist provides certainly has a broader focus. The therapist's coordination of care with other providers heightens his or her awareness of the multilayered nature of the multiple conditions or problems that his or her patient has and allows the therapist to broaden treatment to address these.

Underlying each task is the goal of communicating to patients that the therapist cares about them and that the patients are not alone in the often confusing labyrinth of medical services. While psychotherapists may work to broaden their treatment focus to include preventative care and to act as patient advocates (see Chapter 5), they may encounter resistance from patients. In this case, it is important for therapists to assess each patient's level of motivation and readiness for change.

Resistance, Motivation, and Readiness to Change

Resistance is a concept common to every approach to psychotherapy (Anderson & Stewart, 1983). In fact, many models of therapy have been built around this concept exclusively, and as a result, a substantial and significant body of literature exists on the nature of patient resistance and the therapeutic strategies needed to overcome it.

In medicine, resistance is often discussed in terms of the patient's denial (Ness & Ende, 1994) and noncompliance. While multiple views on resistance depend on one's theoretical orientation, almost every school of therapy recognizes that the patient may have a difficult time changing. Resistance can be viewed as a power struggle between client and therapist, the result of unresolved childhood conflicts, learned negative behaviors, faulty thinking, or numerous other obstacles. Regardless of one's view, it is the professional's responsibility to recognize and address the resistance that the client puts forth.

All approaches to treatment recognize that change, especially significant and lasting change, is hard to achieve and takes time. Perhaps one reason why psychotherapists in traditional practices do not focus much on the prevention of relapses is that they do not see their patients long enough to know whether they relapse or not. Since primary health care is continuous and not limited by treatment of a specific problem, the psychotherapist in a primary care setting can see the patient over time, regardless of the patients' immediate health issues. As a result, preventative care and relapse prevention can become a specific focus of integrated mental health services.

A Model of Change

A practical way of looking at resistance is the transtheoretical model of behavior change originally suggested by Prochaska and DiClemente (1983; Prochaska, Norcross, & DiClemente, 1994). Rather than taking a problem-based focus, which suggests that resistance is something that the clinician must overcome or combat, the transtheoretical model (TTM) facilitates change by building on patient's competencies and focusing on the patient's strengths and resourcefulness. Instead of focusing on the negative qualities of a resistant patient, the clinician using the TTM focuses on the patient's *motivation for change* and the patient's *readiness for change*. This model and its accompanying motivational interviewing strategy have been applied to patients struggling with chemical dependency, smoking cessation, weight management, chronic illness, and a host of other hard-to-change problems Proponents of this model recognize that much of health care depends not on finding the right drug but on helping clients change their daily behaviors. Instead of promoting a miracle cure, Prochaska and colleagues focus on setting manageable goals, helping the client to make small intermediate changes and managing the inevitable lapses.

The TTM contains five stages describing various degrees of readiness to produce change (Prochaska & DiClemente, 1992). Using a stage model helps clinicians see the process of producing change in a series of progressive steps, rather than as an all-or-nothing proposition. It also facilitates the perception that not all patients present to treatment at the same stage of readiness for change. For example, it has been estimated that among any group of people targeted for change, only 20% are ready for action. Forty percent are contemplating change and another 40% are not even thinking about changing. What this means is that treatment plans can and must be developed according to the stage of readiness in which the patient presents. Once the clinician knows the stage of readiness for change, appropriate treatment strategies can be implemented to move the client to the next stage. Treatment essentially involves progressing each patient incrementally through the stages of change and does not include the daunting task of producing change in the resistant patient.

Stages of Change*

Stage 1: *Precontemplation*. Individuals in this stage have not yet begun to even think about change. They may not even recognize that their behavior is problematic. Or they may recognize it as problematic but may not see it as something that affects them or that they need to change.

Stage 2: *Contemplation*. Individuals in this stage are considering making a change. This is a stage of ambivalence in which patients are typically torn between the advantages of changing and the benefits of not changing. People in the contemplation stage are still far from making plans to change.

---

*Prochaska & DiClemente, 1992.

Stage 3: *Preparation.* Individuals in this stage intend to take action and have taken some behavioral steps in this direction.

Stage 4: *Action.* In this stage, individuals begin to initiate change. This is essentially a stage of trying new behaviors.

Stage 5: *Maintenance.* In this stage, individuals have accepted the change and work toward sustaining it.

Motivational Interviewing

Motivational interviewing is a treatment approach based on the TTM (Miller & Rollnick, 1991). According to this approach, the job of the clinician is to identify what stage of the TTM the patient is in and to tailor therapeutic interventions to the patient's level of readiness. Each patient will respond best to interventions that are appropriate to his or her stage of readiness. For example, because a patient in the precontemplation stage does not see that he or she needs to change, the change process is much different from that in someone who is at least considering the possibility of changing. Similarly, it follows that an intervention working with someone in the contemplation stage will most likely not work with someone in the precontemplation stage.

Let's look at what interventions are appropriate at the different stages of readiness. Compared to later stages, patients in the *precontemplation stage* think about their problems less, see less negative consequences to their problem behaviors, and are less responsive to families' and friends' perceptions of their behaviors (Prochaska & DiClemente, 1992). The most appropriate interventions at this stage are consciousness raising and patient education. To move from precontemplation to the contemplation stage, patients must be made aware of the negative consequences of their behaviors—they must feel uncomfortable with them. Often, a meaningful or traumatic personal event or experience such as a laboratory test result or a medical diagnosis will help patients become aware of the negative consequences of their behaviors. However, unplanned personal events do not need to be the only mechanisms to move patients from precontemplation to contemplation. Planned therapeutic strategies that raise consciousness also can be used successfully.

People in the *contemplation stage* are most likely to be receptive to self-evaluation activities. They are in a state of ambivalence—seeing the benefits of changing while at the same time seeing the benefits of not changing. Education, self-help literature, and tasks designed to help them evaluate their goals and values are all successful strategies for moving contemplators to the preparation stage.

Those in the *preparation stage* typically present in treatment with a desire and intent to change but may lack the knowledge, resources, or motivation to carry out the change. Here, the clinician helps patients to make realistic plans for change while appropriately anticipating and planning for potential barriers to change.

Clients often present in the *action stage*, in which they have initiated change but because it is of short duration, it is unable to maintain itself. The action stage typically involves hard work, requiring great cognitive and behavioral effort. Relapsing is not uncommon, and patients should be told this. The clinician's role at this stage is to provide suggestions or strategies for maintaining the change, especially in the face of tendencies toward relapse. Support is particularly important at this stage.

The possibility for relapse still exists for those in the *maintenance stage*. Just as the action stage requires hard work, so does the maintenance stage. Helping patients to evaluate their progress and develop strategies for maintaining the changes they have made is crucial during this stage.

Unique Contributions for the Transtheoretical Model

Another focus of Prochaska and DiClemente's model is rewarding self-control rather than waiting for the environment to provide the reward. Instead of waiting for their clothes size to decrease (environmental reinforcer), dieting patients are told to pick a small reward at the end of the day for maintaining a healthy diet all day. Patients are taught to recognize high-risk situations for relapse, such as holiday parties for the dieting patient. Then they are encouraged to make a plan to prevent relapse during the risky period. "Triggers" for unhealthy living (e.g., eating in front of the television) are identified, and plans are made to avoid the usual unhealthy response.

Many behavioral therapists will recognize similarities between their work and Prochaska and DiClemente's model. However, the focus on self-control versus environmental contingencies, the patient's cognitive state of readiness, and the concept of accepting where a patient is instead of insisting that he or she adhere to the program's standards are all departures from traditional behavioral therapies. Another key difference is the assumption that patients will relapse. Instead of giving up once the relapse occurs, patients are taught to accept themselves and begin working again on their goals to change. Research on smoking cessation, weight loss, and a host of other struggles suggests that maintaining positive changes for a year or two, especially once the program has ended, is one of the most difficult challenges for patients. Thus, maintenance, maintaining the hard-won changes that patients make, is one of the most important areas of research today.

Quality of Life

When health care therapists are working with physicians and their patients, there is usually no shortage of goals, and everyone involved may have slightly different goals. Patients may simply want to "feel better" and be looking for guidance. Physicians might want patients to lower cholesterol level, stop smoking, or lower their anxiety. Therapists hope that patients' anxiety will subside and their work situation will improve (Lynch, Kaplan, & Shema, 1997).

In a collaborative health care setting, how do therapists identify the most important goals or necessary changes? Which factor has the most impact on the patient and how will therapists know if the biopsychosocial interventions have made a difference? To answer these questions, health care specialists have created the concept of health-related quality of life (Wilson & Cleary, 1995). Quality-of-life measures commonly are used in health care settings and medical research but generally are unfamiliar to psychotherapists.

Quality of life has been examined in numerous settings (Kimmel et al., 1995). Quality-of-life variables typically include a person's physical and mental well-being, social support, and existing life stressors. Some researchers include the meaning the patient gives to life as well. These researchers argue that most patients can sustain significant physical and mental hardships with little hope for alleviation as long as they have meaning in their life (Leplege & Hunt, 1997; Wilson & Cleary, 1995).

Kimmel and colleagues (1995) studied the quality of life for hemodialysis patients evaluating the severity of the illness, social support, and psychological well-being. They demonstrated that patient compliance, especially with difficult treatment regimens, is influenced by quality of life. In another study examining mortality after coronary artery bypass graft surgery, researchers found that the physical component of quality of life predicted postoperative mortality while the mental health component did not. Poor scores on the physical health component indicated substantial limitations in self-care; limits in physical, social, and role activities; severe pain; and frequent exhaustion.

In a study examining quality of life for dying patients, managing pain, avoiding inappropriate prolongation of dying, having a sense of control, relieving burden, and strengthening relationships with loved ones were considered important measures of quality of life. A final study looking at the relationships between depression, medical costs, and quality of life (Revicki, Simon, Chan, Keton, & Heiligenstein, 1998) demonstrated that effectively treating depression can improve quality of life.

A key component of these quality-of-life studies is their emphasis on the *patient's subjective report of life* and understanding how each component contributes to the patient's contentment. The patient's report is critical because subjective measures of contentment are not always related to objective measures of life circumstances and functional status, yet the patient's feelings and beliefs about their situation has a significant impact on quality of life (Leplege & Hunt, 1997; Wilson & Cleary, 1995).

While issues surrounding the measurement and conceptualization of quality of life continue to be debated in the health care field, therapists can glean direction from this basic health care concept. They might want to consider to what degree certain illnesses or problems influence a patient's quality of life. For example, one attractive patient in our clinic found out she had terminal breast cancer. All her life she had maintained a strict diet, which included not eating sweets or desserts. Within a month after getting her prognosis, she had gained weight. When queried about this weight gain, she said that she bypassed desserts all her life because she wanted to maintain her appearance. Since she was dying, she saw little reason to deny herself the small pleasure of eating desserts.

The quality-of-life concept is helpful in thinking about patients for several reasons. First, it helps therapists to examine the multitude of influences that affect a patient's feeling about life. For example, it helps them understand how a patient with debilitating chronic pain but strong family support and strong coping skills can continue to prosper while another patient with a nominal health concern can function poorly in day-to-day life. It also helps therapists to think beyond the traditional therapy goals such as alleviating the patient's depression or treating agoraphobia.

In addition, thinking about the patient's view of quality of life helps therapists to understand what is important to the patient. This information can help them set target goals that will motivate the client to pursue potentially difficult treatments as well as encourage patient compliance. Lastly, quality of life helps therapists to know what the baseline is and thus set realistic goals. For example, a patient with serious chronic pain and underlying psychopathology can have an improved life but perhaps not as satisfying as the patient with no psychopathology or illness.

Specific Problems

Health care organizations are greatly interested in assessing the value of educational and preventative care, and it follows that there is no shortage of opinions about its worth. Viewing preventative care as a critical part of the health care system with regards to keeping costs down and increasing health, Rosenthal (1997, p. 1) asserted that "investing in preventive care is a cornerstone of our business because of the tremendous returns it provides. It keeps health care costs low by preventing serious illness and promoting a healthy lifestyle." At the other extreme, Rosenthal (1997) wrote that "if you are a company looking at what gives you a return on your investment, immunizations certainly have a payoff, and smoking cessation in pregnant women is probably also a slam dunk. Beyond that, our conversation is over. That's it" (p. 1). As these differences in opinion point out, the measures one uses to assess preventative care influence the results.

Although preventative care may not ultimately save health care dollars, it is an important benefit to employers and employees who are purchasing health care services. Because it is difficult to quantify the actual savings to the health care organization, one must look beyond cost and marketability and turn to a third important measure, the health and well-being of patients. Using patients' well-being as the yardstick, preventative care programs are excellent investments.

In this section, we briefly review some sample problems and the educational programs that address these problems. Various treatment programs have been found to be effective in each of these areas; however, in this brief section, we simply introduce therapists to some options that their primary care patients may have. Therapists who do not feel comfortable addressing preventative issues with clients can help locate effective resources to ameliorate these problems. They can then coordinate their treatment plans in conjunction with these programs.

Eating, Weight, and Physical Exercise

Recent large-scale studies on obesity in the United States indicated that between one-fourth to one-half of all Americans are obese and that the incidence of obesity is increasing (Mokdad et al., 1999; Must et al., 1999). From 1991 to 1998, the incidence of obesity increased in every state, in both sexes, and across all age groups, races, educational levels, and smoking status. Obese patients face an increased risk of diabetes mellitus, gallbladder disease, coronary heart disease, high blood cholesterol level, high blood pressure, and osteoarthritis. Despite the fact that these illnesses are often fatal, more people are becoming more obese every year.

This trend of more Americans gaining more weight every year is surprising considering American culture. As one of our adolescent patients said, "Thin is in." Americans look at fat content on food containers as they go down grocery store aisles picking out food. They often live near several gyms or have exercise equipment available through their work or at home. They purchase jogging equipment or query their physicians about weight loss medication. Popular magazines in racks at the grocery store checkout line tout yet another miracle diet. In spite of this focus on weight and physical appearance, Americans continue to grow larger.

In a study examining the prevalence of attempted weight loss, Serdula and colleagues (1999) point out that one third to one half of all Americans are attempting to lose weight. The most common weight loss strategy was to consume less fat but not fewer calories. A small percentage of those patients trying to lose weight follow a recommended combination of eating fewer calories and engaging in physical activity. These findings suggest that inquiring about weight-loss goals and providing diet education could help patients lose weight, thus preventing the numerous health risks associated with being overweight.

While many patients' efforts to lose weight are misguided and ultimately fail, there are proven programs that prevent future health problems such as coronary heart disease (Boyle, O'Connor, Pronk, & Tan, 1998). For example the work by Ornish and colleagues (1998) on the "Lifestyle Heart Trial" led to reversal of coronary heart disease. Recent research also suggests that adherence to a lifestyle of health eating, weekly exercise, and abstinence from smoking is associated with a very low risk of coronary heart disease (Stampfer et al., 2000).

Evidence suggesting that patients want to lose weight but are unsure about what to do suggests that physicians should be actively involved in their patients' weight and diet concerns. However, recent research indicated that most physicians do not recommend a weight loss or exercise program to their overweight patients (Galuska, Will, Serdula, & Ford, 1999). In one study, less than half of obese adults reported being advised to lose weight by their physician (Galuska et al., 1999). This is surprising since patients whose physicians suggested a weight loss program were three times more likely to undertake such a program. Even among patients who did receive a recommendation from their physician, only half had used the recommended strategy of combining diet and physical activity.

Physicians may selectively choose whom to counsel about weight loss and exercise. Patients more likely to be counseled include overweight, educated, middle-aged women, particularly those who have diabetes. Patients of lower socioeconomic status, men, young people, and patients only slightly overweight are less likely to be counseled about weight control or exercise.

There are few data on how much therapists bring up weight loss and physical activity with clients. Perhaps many therapists believe that these areas are outside their scope of practice. However, there is growing evidence that physical activity can physiologically influence depressive symptoms (Wang, 2001). In addition, most people's feelings about their weight influence their sense of well-being and self-esteem.

From a biopsychosocial perspective, ignoring weight or physical activity when treating problems like depression or anxiety is tantamount to the biomedical specialist ignoring the patient's emotions about his or her physical illness. Therapists are trained to inquire about substance abuse or suicide risk regardless of whether the patient brings it up. In similar fashion, therapists can inquire about the patient's feelings and initiatives about weight and physical activity.

Perhaps therapists are reluctant to ask about weight issues, fearing that they will offend their patient. Working in a medical setting may provide a foray into these difficult subjects. In addition, explaining to the patient their biopsychosocial philosophy helps the patient understand that therapists are looking at his or her whole life and that they see the interconnections rather than simply focusing on traditional mental health concerns.

There are numerous weight loss programs available, each with a slightly different focus. However, almost all weight loss programs include the following components:

1. learning to eat a healthy diet
2. doing at least moderate exercise (such as rapid walking) at least three times a week
3. receiving social support, either from groups, family members, coaches, or trainers
4. learning to recognize triggers for overeating
5. coping with lapses

Therapists can learn what programs are available through their clients' health plans. Some patients want aggressive programs such as liquid diets or medication to lose weight. Others simply want to shed the five pounds that they gained over the holidays. Regardless, therapists should be open to working with clients on their weight and physical activity along with their more traditional mental health concerns. It is simply a matter of asking.

Sleep Problems

Everyone experiences sleeplessness sometime during their life. People under-stand that worry or stressful life circumstances can temporarily interrupt sleep. However, approximately one-third of the population has a more serious sleep dis-turbance during their lifetime. The most common symptoms patients report is feeling drowsy when awake (Ancoli-Israel, 1996; Maorin, 1993).

Primary care providers including the mental health professional not only must diagnose the sleep problem but also must understand the etiology. Common sleeping problems seen in primary care include insomnia, hypersomnia, irregular breathing, narcolepsy, periodic limb movement during sleep, and parasomnias. *Narcolepsy* refers to an irresistible urge to sleep during the day. *Periodic limb move-ment* refers to twitching or jerking of the limbs, usually the legs, every few seconds. *Parasomnias* refer to intense physical experiences that happen during sleep such as night terrors, sleepwalking, and nightmares (Ancoli-Israel, 1996). Insomnia increases with age and is more common in women and in lower socioe-conomic classes. Other disorders such as snoring are more common in men, espe-cially overweight men (Rakel, 1993).

Complaints about sleep problems sometimes mask underlying or co-existing problems. For example, depression, anxiety, and substance abuse problems com-monly co-occur with sleep problems. Many sleep-deprived patients have serious psychosocial stressors such as threatened job loss or concurrent physical illness. Sleep problems are associated with greater functional impairment, lost produc-tivity, and excess health care utilization (Simon & Von Korff, 1997). Insomnia and other sleep problems are often not treated effectively in primary care (Shochat, Umphress, & Ancoli-Israel, 1999).

Physical or mental health problems frequently are associated with sleep prob-lems. In fact, there are a variety of causes (Ancoli-Israel, 1996), including :

- behavioral factors (e.g., taking afternoon naps)
- medical factors (e.g., as a symptom of dementia)
- psychiatric causes (e.g., as a symptom of anxiety or depression)
- drugs (e.g., drinking alcohol or taking a stimulant including caffeine or decongestants)
- circadian rhythm disturbances (e.g., jet lag)
- disorders (e.g., sleep apnea, narcolepsy)

An instrument that can be used to assess sleep is the Stanford Sleepiness Scale that examines how alert, drowsy, or sleepy the patient is (Hoddes, Zarcone,

Smythe, Phillips, & Dement, 1973). Another common primary care assessment tool is a sleep diary kept by the patient. In addition, most physicians include questions about sleep-related problems as part of their clinical interview.

Sleep loss may be the patient's primary concern, but often, especially when there are other physical or mental health problems, changes in sleep are described as a symptom of a larger problem. In some cases, the patient may be so used to the sleep problem and so consumed by other symptoms such as worry or sadness that he or she fails to mention sleep disturbances. Thus, it is essential that the clinician remember to ask about changes in sleep.

In other situations, sleep issues may never arise in the discussion—either as a cause or as a problem. For example, one of us knows a pediatrician whose first question when evaluating for attention deficit disorder is, "How many hours of sleep does this child get per night?" The physician believes that for years he was "treating" attention problems that were really concentration and fatigue problems resulting from too little sleep. In general, children of all ages and teenagers receive significantly less sleep than they need. These sleep-deprived children may show symptoms of inattention, irritability, volatility, and inability to concentrate. Instead of focusing on the sleep deprivation, the therapist inadvertently focuses on the symptoms of the sleep deprivation.

Most mental health professionals other than psychiatrists are trained to view sleep disturbance as a symptom of a disorder but not to do a more careful assessment or to treat the sleep problem. Perhaps it is believed that when the primary symptom (e.g., worry, sadness, guilt, fear) abates, the sleep problem will be cured. This is one more situation where mental health therapists working in a health care setting can expand their professional identity and implement a biopsychosocial model.

While the focus of treatment may be on treating the psychosocial concerns, therapists can still suggest simple treatments. For example, cognitive behavioral theory provides several suggestions in response to common behavioral sleep problems. The two most common behavioral sleep problems are fear about not being able to sleep and poor sleep hygiene (or bad sleep habits). The basic recommendations of good sleep hygiene include:

1. Curtail time in bed.
2. Get up at the same time each day.
3. Avoid the bedroom clock.
4. Avoid caffeine, alcohol, and tobacco.
5. Exercise.
6. Eat a light snack.

7. Adjust the sleeping environment so that it is peaceful and dark.
8. Do not worry right before bed.

In addition to providing suggestions for good sleep hygiene, the mental health provider can teach the patient biofeedback techniques and relaxation skills, such as meditation and breathing exercises. Cognitive behavioral therapies address and try to change some of the beliefs patients have about their sleep (Morin, 1993). Some mental health therapists are trained in special sleep treatments including stimulus-control therapy and sleep restriction therapy (Bootzin & Perlis, 1992; Spielman, Saskin, & Thorpy, 1987; Baillargeon, 1997). Box 8.1 provides guidelines for these two sleep treatment therapies.

Beside behavioral therapies that the mental health professional can offer, the physician has the option of prescribing a sleep medication. Some new types of drugs have resulted in more positive effects (e.g., deeper sleep) and fewer negative side effects (e.g., residual daytime drowsiness, rebound insomnia when the drugs are stopped, and development of tolerance). Nevertheless pharmacological treatment should be aimed at the underlying disorders such as depression, anxiety, and pain. Physicians frequently recommend that sleeping pills should be used for relief of symptoms and should not be used for more than a few weeks at a time. In addition, they tell patients that medications should not be taken with alcohol and should be given at the lowest possible effective dose.

Common Problems

As mentioned earlier, it is beyond the scope of this book to discuss all of the excellent current literature available on common mental disorders in health care settings or methods of prevention. However, we would like to briefly mention several more issues that commonly arise in primary care settings and could be the focus of prevention efforts by the mental health professional.

Child and Adolescent Problems (Including Child Abuse)

Mental health problems in children and adolescents frequently go unrecognized and remain untreated. Problems such as attention deficit disorder, pervasive developmental disorders, and anxiety disorders are commonly seen in pediatrics or family medicine. Parents and school personnel may recognize that something is awry with the child's development but have no idea what to do. Often, overwhelmed parents look first to their primary care providers for help.

Box 8.1
Guidelines for Two Sleep Treatment Therapies

STIMULUS-CONTROL THERAPY

This therapy attempts to break the negative cycles of being in bed but unable to sleep (Bootzin & Perlis, 1992). The rules of stimulus-control therapy include

1. Only go to bed when you feel sleepy.
2. If you don't fall asleep within 15 minutes, get out of bed. Stay out of bed until you can fall asleep.
3. Avoid looking at the clock.
4. Get up at the same time every morning
5. Use the bed only for sleeping, not for watching TV, reading, or doing paperwork.
6. Do not nap during the day.

SLEEP-RESTRICTION THERAPY

This therapy is based on the idea that too much time spent in bed leads to poor sleep (Spielman et al., 1987). Guidelines for sleep-restriction therapy include

1. You are allowed to stay in bed only for the amount of time you are sleeping plus 15 minutes.
2. You must get up at the same time every day.
3. Do not nap during the day.
4. When you are asleep for 85% of the time you are in bed, you can increase the amount of time in bed by going to bed 15 minutes earlier.
5. Repeat this process until you are sleeping for eight hours.

In one study, researchers demonstrated that a prenatal program and early-childhood home visitation by nurses to high-risk families reduced the incidence of adolescent antisocial behavior and substance abuse 15 years later (Olds et al., 1998). In the accompanying editorial, the editors stated that "early intervention can produce positive and persistent change in human development and also strengthen the base of knowledge regarding the nature of infant vulnerabilities and the hazards . . . faced from substandard living environments" (Olds et al., 1998, p. 1271).

Another area of prevention is the recognition of child abuse. While many mental health professionals have some training in child abuse recognition, it is still easily overlooked in a health care setting. While Kempe, Silverman, Steele, Droegemueller, and Silver's classic article (1962) on "the battered child" changed the field of child abuse forever, recent research suggested that health care professionals are still frequently missing indicators of abuse (Carole, Hymel, Ritzen, Reinert, & Hay, 1999; Jenny, 1999; Leventhal, 1999).

It is easy to overlook the needs of children and adolescents in busy health care settings, even pediatric practices, if the demands are so great that the physician only has time to address the immediate concerns in a 15-minute visit. One of us was asked to consult with a physician about an anxious, depressed woman whose alcoholic husband had dropped dead in front of her during the previous week. She was working a night shift and had little money. She reported that she was ambivalent about his death because their relationship had been violent and abusive. The physician and therapist spent 30 minutes talking to the patient about her life situation. During the last five minutes of the office visit, she casually mentioned that she was also concerned about her two young adolescents who had witnessed the violence, the substance abuse, and their father's death. She left them home alone at night when she went to work. Their sleep had become disrupted by nightmares after their father's death and she wondered aloud what she might do to help them with their nightmares.

The needs of these children could easily have been completely missed. As it was, the physician had to move on to the next patient. Yet the therapist was able to schedule a visit the next day to do a more complete family assessment and plan. Over the next few months, the primary care providers offered critical support and suggestions for the family.

Violence

Violence in the United States runs the risk of becoming endemic. Each year approximately 25,500 people die from homicide and 31,000 die from suicide (Rosenberg et al., 1997). Violence is associated with substance abuse, child abuse and neglect, and a multitude of psychological problems and physical symptoms throughout the victim's life (McCauley et al., 1997).

Nevertheless, violence often goes unrecognized in health care settings (Rodriguez, Bauer, McLoughlin, & Grumbach, 1999). In addition, battered women report that their physicians can be insensitive during their interviews (Hamberger,

Ambuel, Marbella, & Donze, 1998). Common complaints include the provider treating the physical injuries but not asking how they happened. If the symptoms of violence are recognized during a medical visit, the patient is often referred to a mental health professional. Recognizing sysmptoms of violence is a critical first step in the prevention of violence.

Three brief questions can be used to screen for violence (Feldhaus, 1997):

1. Have you been hit, kicked, punched, or otherwise hurt by someone within the past year?
2. Do you feel safe in your current relationship?
3. Is there a partner from a previous relationship who is making you feel unsafe now?

A collaborative model for assessment and treatment of violence offers the needed resources to address this biopsychosocial problem. The biological results—bruises, broken bones, head injuries—can be addressed more easily than the psychosocial precursors. In addition, addressing violence can often feel overwhelming and confusing to health care providers. A team approach offers the necessary resources to address this complex and growing epidemic.

Stress

A rich body of literature exists on the impact of stress on physical health including discussions about acute stressors (a sudden death of a loved one), chronic stressors (caring for a disabled family member), and pile-up of stressors (caring for an ill family member that leads to financial crises, social isolation, and overwhelming emotions). This literature suggests that distress occurs when environmental demands exceed a person's ability to adapt or cope.

The resulting distress places the person at higher risk for diseases, especially cardiovascular and infectious illnesses. Even if the person does not become physically ill, he or she is likely to have some physical symptoms as a result of the stress. Headaches, inability to sleep, muscle fatigue, and exhaustion are common complaints resulting from stress. At times, the person may decide that their physical symptoms warrant a visit to the physician.

As we have mentioned earlier, researchers are only beginning to understand the physiological links between psychosocial variables such as anger, frustration, and sadness and physical health. We do know that stressors such as job loss, a change in health status, or relationship problems can change parts of the cellular immune responses. Stressors and the patient's emotional responses to stress affect immune functioning by disrupting the nervous, endocrine, and immune systems (Glasser et al., 1999; Gullette et al., 1997; McEwen, 1998).

Mental health providers working in health care settings are in unique positions to address the effects of stress and the antidotes. This need not involve extensive therapy. Allowing the patient to express emotions, change the way they are thinking about a problem, discover new solutions to stressors, and setting new lifestyle goals are ways that therapists can do brief, effective interventions. Glaser and colleagues suggest "there is reason to think that certain changes in lifestyle might increase . . . resistance to infectious diseases. These include broadening one's social involvements (e.g., joining social or spiritual groups, having a confidant, spending time with supportive friends) and being more careful to maintain healthful practices such as proper diet, exercise, and sleep" (p. 2270).

The first step to treating stress is to recognize it. This can be difficult when patients only complain about physical symptoms and do not mention the challenging events in their lives. The presence of a mental health expert in the physician's office may help remind the physician to ask about the patient's personal circumstances. Some patients make the link between their life events and physical symptoms themselves. Regardless of how it happens, recognizing the effects of stress, especially when they present only as physical symptoms, is a key first step.

If the patient chooses to work with a mental health expert, the treatment is usually focused and brief. Sometimes we will simply make a list of the stressors the patient faces. Making this list can be an effective intervention because it can help the patient realize for the first time the many challenges they face. After making the list, we explore possible solutions for each stressor.

During these discussions, we can serve as a resource consultant. We try to keep up with community resources and make them available to our patients. For example, we know of volunteer in-home care services for patients caring for disabled family members. These services allow the caregiver a few hours of respite. We also know about Internet sites and chat rooms that address specific stressors. We often explore spiritual resources that the patient might have. These resources may be internal, such as a personal faith or belief system, or external, a church or temple that has meetings, education facilities, or other resources.

At times, we also realize the chronic nature of the stressful event. For example, a terminally ill family member whose illness is progressive, prolonged unemployment, an unwanted divorce or some other experience where the patient has little control over the situation. In these instances, we simply try to provide some support and relief. Recognizing our own limits, we hope that our ongoing interest offers some solace to our patients.

Smoking

It has long been known that the single most preventable cause of disease and death is cigarette smoking (Goldstein et al., 1998; Murphy & Sciandra, 1983). Despite the much publicized attempts by tobacco company executives to hide this fact in the mid- and late 1990s, the medical community has long known the damaging effects of long-term smoking, both in the cause of disease and in the exacerbation of symptoms. In fact, in 1964 the Surgeon General's Advisory Committee Report on smoking identified the etiological connection between smoking and a variety of diseases, including cancer, coronary artery disease, and chronic obstructive pulmonary disease (Terry, 1983). This alarming report was generated as a result of over 25 years of growing scientific concern about the negative effects of cigarette smoking! It is not surprising that medical costs for smokers are quite high. For example, in 1993 medical expenditures related to smoking topped $50 billion for that year alone (Centers for Disease Control, 1994), and there is evidence that medical visits by smokers are 4.3 times higher than the national average (Wetzler & Cruess, 1985).

Concerns about smoking have continued to be voiced unceasingly from within the medical community, with data continuing to point to the deleterious effects of cigarette smoking on health, not only for the smoker but also for those who are around the smoker. Serious health-related consequences of maternal smoking on the fetus, in addition to consequences of secondhand smoke on family members living in the same household (particularly children) as well as coworkers, have been identified.

The result of these data has been the passage of laws throughout the United States that make it illegal to smoke in public buildings and many public places. California, which is probably the most progressive of states when it comes to smoking legislation, has even made it illegal to smoke in restaurants and bars. However, these laws have not come without resistance. In fact, not until recently have substantial decreases in smoking behavior been noted, and these decreases have only been observed within specific population groups and regions of the country. It is interesting that despite the overwhelming evidence suggesting the negative health-related consequences of smoking, the American public, including physicians, continues to be resistant to "giving up the habit."

Smoking reached its peak in 1981, with the actual number of smokers greater than at any other time in history. Since then the number of smokers in the general population has plateaued and recently has decreased (Hymowitz et al., 1991). In the past, during the heyday of smoking, most smokers were white males. In fact, it was estimated that in the late 1940s more than 70% of American males between the ages of 20 and 30 were smokers (Hymowitz, Sexton, Ockene, & Grandits, 1991; Warner, 1986).

In spite of the fact that there has been an overall decrease in the number of smokers over the past 20 years, the demographics of smoking has changed considerably. Most notably, while there has been a noticeable decrease in the number of white male smokers, there has been an alarming increase in the number of African American and female smokers. In fact, the prevalence of smoking among African Americans, especially African American males, is now higher than for whites (Allen, Pederson, & Leonard, 1998). These are distressing statistics, given that the rates of lung cancer and coronary artery disease, conditions for which smoking is an etiological factor, are also higher in African Americans than in whites (Allen, Pederson, & Leonard, 1998; Devesa & Diamond, 1983; Hymowitz et al., 1991; Sempos, Cooper, Kovar, & McMillan, 1988). An increase in smoking among women also has been noted, with women now equally likely to smoke as men. In fact, teenage girls are more likely to begin smoking, and at an earlier age, than teenage boys. Although the reasons for the changing demographics of smoking are unclear, it may have to do with the targeting of males through prevention and cessation programs and the targeting of African Americans and women through cigarette advertising.

Given the preponderance of evidence suggesting the harmful health effects of smoking, there have been a large number of prevention and cessation initiatives, which generally have been met with success. Also, probably because most smokers report that they want to quit (CDC, 1997), even minimal intervention by physicians can be successful. For example, one study found that brief physician advice and encouragement resulted in a quit rate of 2% at 12 months after the intervention (Law & Tang, 1995). Given that this brief encounter with the physician was that only advice and encouragement received by that provider and the extremely high relapse rate with smoking cessation (Hymowitz et al., 1991), this is an impressive percentage. Other studies of physician advice have found similar success rates and these rates are improved when coupled with nicotine replacement therapies (Hurt et al., 1994).

Despite these success rates, not all physicians counsel smoking patients to quit. Goldstein and colleagues (1998) conducted a survey of physicians practicing in Rhode Island and found that 67% of physicians report that they ask about the smoking behavior of their patients and 74% report that they advise their patients about the health risks involved with smoking. Although it is comforting to know that most physicians ask and advise their patients about smoking behavior, it is disconcerting to learn that 26 to 33% do not ask and advise. This is even more disturbing given the suspicion that physicians are likely to overestimate the degree to which they talk to their patients about smoking behavior (Goldstein et al., 1998). Even more disconcerting is that the study found that only 35% of their respondents reported that they help their patients in smoking cessation and a discouraging 8% arrange follow-up visits with their smoking patients to check on progress.

The Goldstein study also found that unaffiliated physicians practicing in private offices were more likely to report being active in attempting to help their patients quit smoking than were physicians affiliated with a managed care practice. They also found that internal medicine physicians were most likely to report higher involvement in smoking cessation and that obstetrician/gynecologists were least likely of all the primary care specialty groups.

Although it is uncertain why affiliated physicians are less likely to work with patients on smoking cessation, as Goldstein and colleagues (1998) pointed out, it may be that physicians working in managed care settings have time demands and productivity requirements that discourage their involvement in smoking cessation counseling. It may also be that the emphasis on patient education and preventative medicine common in managed care settings relieves physicians of their role in patient education about the risks of smoking. Physicians in these settings may believe that patients are getting this advice from other members of the health care team. Regardless of the reasons, physicians within these settings are less likely to counsel patients on the dangers of smoking than are other physicians.

This is precisely where psychotherapists working within these facilities may be of help. Therapists working with patients who smoke can inquire about their smoking and their desires to quit. Therapists can discuss these findings with the physician responsible for their medical care and point patients in the direction of receiving cessation counseling.

Chapter 9

Integrated Health Care—A New Horizon for Psychotherapists

The changing health care environment provides exciting new opportunities for mental health professionals. We have a rare opportunity to be part of a major social shift in how health care is provided and to influence how this shift occurs. We can be at the table reaffirming that patient's needs and feelings remain priorities as systems and services are redesigned. Our identity and roles will also expand and change while we interact with the influences outside the clinical hour that shape health care delivery.

Mental health clinicians who enter the health care field conscious of the broad mission of medical care will likely find themselves being heartily welcomed by medical clinicians and clinics. Mental health and medical providers, once starting down the path together, linked by a common mission to provide the total care their patients need, can develop long-term collaborative relationships that rarely develop in the traditional separate and parallel systems of care.

These collaborative relationships can be harnessed not only for better patient care, but also for the transformation of the care system. This is the greater task, as the clinical insights about integrated care most often exceed the organizational capacities to carry it out. It takes partnership between medical and mental health clinicians and leaders who see themselves as part of a larger professional community with a mission that includes them both, and who see themselves working on the same side of a larger struggle to transform health care in this important way. The energy that flows between people when this partnership occurs can carry the work through the inevitable adversity and challenges, and sustain their vision of health care.

Throughout this book, our aim was to map out ways of crossing the chasm between mental and medical health care and to bridge the gap created by separate and parallel systems of care. We close by highlighting some of the opportunities for therapists to influence the system of care as well as take care of patients.

Mental health professionals in medical care settings are well suited for a consulting role to care teams. In a consultant role, the mental health clinician shifts from being solely responsible for a stand-alone mental health treatment process to being a facilitator who shares his or her expertise with the treatment team and helps organize the system of care. The mental health professional can act not only on behalf of the patient, but on behalf of the aspirations of clinic, the doctors, or the medical group in which he or she works.

Mental health professionals can facilitate resolution of cultural differences between medical and mental health professionals. Mental health professionals can make transparent what used to occur in the provervial "black box" of therapy, help resolve differences in norms for confidentiality and team-based information sharing, and differences in work style and customs. Mental health professionals can join efforts to improve the care system they work in, as a way of improving quality of care and of improving clinic life for clinicians and staff. Mental health clinicians may wonder at times who their clients are—the physicians they are assisting, managers who expect them to provide consistent and understandable treatments at a reasonable cost, employers, family members, schools or courts who may have an interest in the patient, or the patients themselves. In reality, therapists and all clinicians live and work in a world of multiple perspectives. Along with the challenge of balancing these comes the opportunity to develop other sides of the therapists skill set as "systems thinker".

The mental health clinician's role as patient advocate can be strengthened. There may be situations in which the therapist can help the patient resolve misunderstandings or dissatisfactions with their primary care doctor. The therapist can work with the patient to constructively bring up his or her concerns with their physician rather than continue "sitting on feelings or concerns" or begin a journey of seeking out the "perfect physician." In all of these challenging situations the therapist plays a vital role in both changing the care delivered while simultaneously helping the patient successfully navigate the health care system.

Working in the medical setting expands the mental health clinician's knowledge base. Mental health professionals may be initially frustrated about their lack of understanding of the biological parts of the biopsychosocial model, especially if their patients know more about the idiosyncrasies of their illnesses than they do. With each new patient rapid learning takes place as the patient can become an excellent teacher to the mental health professional in learning about the etiology and course of a patient's illness. The most common ways that therapists learn the basic scientific knowledge to understand the illness is to ask the physician questions, read medical literature and do Internet searches. Therapists in medical settings will also learn about basic health practice such as sleep, exercise, eating/diet, and immune functioning. Understanding the biological facts of health, illness, and their treatments, including knowledge about brain functioning and psychotropic medications is also an important part of the therapist's knowledge base.

While therapists are typically trained on suicide assessment, they will quickly add to their "crisis repetoire" how to handle situations such as the patient discovering he has HIV/AIDS, cancer, or other life-threatening illness. Several problem areas that a therapist in a medical setting will become knowledgeable about include end-of-life-care, chronic illness, HIV, somatization, and nebulous illnesses such as chronic fatigue syndrome.

Mental health professionals will be pleasantly surprised by the positive treatment outcomes that can occur with brief interventions. Therapists in medical settings begin to think about treatment as short-term instead of long-term. Models of short-term therapy have emerged in the mental health fields, but most of these still imply four to eight visits. In the medical setting, we've learned that short-term can mean one visit, and this visit may last no more than 15 minutes. Ultimately, this means that treatment duration is moving from a traditional 50-minute hour to doing whatever the patient and physician needs.

Mental health professionals will benefit from the enhanced impact of practicing as part of the primary care team. Mental health professionals may feel some loss of independent practice autonomy in a medical setting. However, most feel well rewarded by the benefits of interdisciplinary collegiality and the ability to get more done for patients. These benefits include the opportunity to learn from other disciplines. Instead of viewing professionals from other disciplines as a potential threat for control, which occurs in the traditional fragmented care system, these professionals are part of a team and are valued for what they can bring to the table when discussing patient care.

It is a source of pride and satisfaction to see all the disciplines touching the patient's life as a combined effort, with the mental health services being one facet.

Appendix A

Dissatisfaction with Fragmented Medical and Mental Health Care*

Examples of Common Clinician Dissatisfactions

1. Knowledge about the patient is limited.
   - Several charts, each providing just one piece of the story.
   - Charts are missing.

2. Contacting other clinicians for additional information is laborious and impractical.
   - Efforts to contact another provider results in "phone tag."
   - If you are a primary care physician, the therapist cannot talk to you, due to confidentiality issues.
   - Practices and schedules are set up to expedite referrals, not to expedite talking about cases.

3. Making referrals between primary care and behavioral health care can be an adventure.
   - If you are a primary care physician, it is difficult to engage patients about behavioral health factors related to their physical problems.
     - ❏ Behavioral health referrals have to be "sold" to patients who view their problems as medical.
     - ❏ You have little knowledge of the behavioral health providers.

*Appendix A is based on the experiences of C. J. Peek and R. L. Heinrich, and is adapted from Peek & Heinrich, 2000, with permission of Lawrence Erlbaum Associates.

❏ You receive limited behavioral health feedback.
- If you are a behavioral health professional,
  ❏ Patients may only come in because of a physician referral.
  ❏ Physicians often tell patients what the behavioral health outcome will be, and often times, the projected outcome doesn't fit.

4. Many patient problems do not fit into separated medical or behavioral health domains.
- It is a challenge to address emotional factors that might contribute to headache or lower back pain in a 15-minute visit.
- Somatization is common and difficult to address effectively using an either-or approach to medical and behavioral health care.
- Distress and adjustment problems frequently arise in families coping with chronic illnesses.
- Some patients keep coming back even when physicians have nothing left to offer.
- Mental health providers may not know how to respond to patients' physical problems.

Examples of Common Patient Dissatisfactions

1. "I am physically ill but they think it's all in my head."
- "I do not need to receive behavioral health care, I have a medical problem."
- "I realize my emotions affect my health, but my physical problem is not only a psychological symptom."

2. "When will someone ask about how my family life and problems are affecting my health?"
- "Living like this must have something to do with my physical problems."

3. "I have a family doctor, a specialist, a psychiatrist, a therapist, and a group therapist. Do they talk to each other?"
- "They keep sending me from one person to the next!"
- "I tell the same story over and over to each new person."
- "Why don't they talk to each other!"
- "No wonder health insurance is so high!"

4. "It seems like I see doctors all the time, but I'm still not getting better."
   - "I get the feeling I am not being a good patient."
   - "I get the feeling no one wants to see me anymore."
   - "It seems like they are trying to cut me off."
   - "I get the feeling everything is my fault."

Examples of Common Care System Dissatisfactions

1. Utilization of outpatient visits is high and unfocused.
   - When delivery services do not match clinical needs, searching and unnecessary visits result.
   - Disability management is a major, but often underaddressed, behavioral issue across most medical diseases.

2. Hospital and referral costs are unnecessarily high.
   - Narrower understanding of the patient and family leaves clinicians and families with fewer options.
   - Patient is referred or hospitalized when a break in continuity or coordination of care occurs at the wrong time.

3. Patients are often unhappy with care, even though they get a lot of it.
   - Some of these patients become "difficult"; most difficult patients started out merely as complex.
   - Patients are trying to secure help by shopping for physicians.

4. Misunderstandings occur between primary care and behavioral health providers.
   - There is a limited understanding of what different professions can contribute to the total care of patients.
   - Pejorative mutual stereotypes are based on limited contact and opportunity to work out problems.

5. The problems of separate and parallel medical and mental health care are no longer acceptable as a normal cost of doing business.
   - Care systems can no longer postpone redesigning basic care processes to improve total system quality.
   - Care systems can no longer afford the satisfaction and service penalties associated with fragmented care.

- Care systems can no longer absorb the unnecessary financial costs associated with fragmented care.
- Care systems must meet new National Committee on Quality Assurance (NCQA) standards for primary care–behavioral health integration.

Examples of Employer Dissatisfaction

1. Traditional behavioral health care is often seen as an expense of dubious value.
   - It is a "black hole" where employees and benefit dollars often disappear.
   - Therapies often do not emphasize the value to patients of good work adjustment; instead, they are often preoccupied with abstract and impractical psychological matters.
   - Therapies do not have the needs of employers in mind, such as getting people back to work or becoming more productive and less absorbed with their personal problems.

2. Employers experience productivity or behavior problems with the employees they suspect have mental health or substance abuse issues, but who will not seek behavioral health care.
   - Employers are aware that employee distress and health problems do not sort themselves neatly into traditional behavioral health and medical categories.
   - Employers know that primary care is the de facto mental health system.
   - Employers know that psychologically distressed patients are not only more expensive employees, but also more costly in terms of health care benefits.

3. Employers experience productivity problems attributable to family and marital distress that are not covered by benefits but add to medical and employer costs.
   - Family and marital distress are usually excluded from mental health benefits but often adversely affect productivity, other employees, supervisors, and employer costs.
   - Many employers are already paying additional costs for employee assistance programs (EAPs) to cover noncovered psychosocial problems.

4. Employers have to deal with employees complaining about fragmentation in the care system.
   - Benefit managers hear complaints about fragmentation and poor service in the care system.
   - Benefit managers are asked to intervene for employees by asking for exceptions to benefits because the covered services do not match clinical needs.

Appendix B

Components of the Biopsychosocial Model

Biomedical Information

Engel (1980) listed several requirements necessary to implement a biopsychoso-cial model. One requirement is biomedical information such as laboratory data, which can indicate the presence of a disease that the patient does not realize he or she has. For example, diabetes and schizophrenia are two diseases that may be present biochemically but are unknown to the patient. Kaplan (2000) recognized this growing phenomenon by talking about a "disease reservoir"—the idea that each person carries a multitude of latent diseases that may or may not become symptomatic. At what point in this process does the patient "have the illness"?

Engel's recognition of this phenomenon predates the exploding knowledge of the human genome project. In the future, patients may know years before its actual occurrence that there is a good probability a life-threatening illness will develop. If genetic testing suggests a patient is likely to get breast cancer, but she is com-pletely asymptomatic at that time, except for clinical depression that develops in response to this information, how should we view her health/disease dilemmas?

Interviewing Skills

Another essential requirement to implement a biopsychosocial model is inter-viewing skills that match the specificity of technical and laboratory procedures. Engel stated that "the most essential skills of the physician involve the ability to elicit accurately and then analyze correctly the patient's verbal account of his illness experience. . . . The biomedical model ignores both the rigor required to achieve reliability in the interview process and the necessity to analyze the meaning of the patient's report in psychological, social and cultural as well as in anatomical, physiological, or biochemical terms" (Engel, 1992a, p. 323).

Knowledge of the Patient's Environment

Knowledge of the patient's environment is another essential criterion. By now, it is well documented that variables such as stress and social isolation can significantly influence both the course and the onset of an illness (Selye, 1976; Kiecold-Glaser & Glaser, 1995).

Understanding the Meaning That the Patient Gives to the Biochemical Process

Understanding the meaning that the patient gives to the biochemical process is also a critical part of a biopsychosocial model (Wright et al., 1998). For example, an unanticipated pregnancy may be one of the peak life experiences for an infertile couple who had resigned themselves to being childless. On the other hand, for a poor, single woman who already has two children, an unanticipated pregnancy may be one of the biggest crises of her life. The same physiological experience has two distinct meanings depending on each patient's viewpoint and context.

Respect for That Which Cannot be Tested

A final ingredient of the biopsychosocial model is respect for that which cannot be tested—the spiritual and unexplained parts of the human response to illness and pain. Engel (1977, p. 328) suggested that "general systems theory provides a conceptual approach suitable for a biopsychosocial concept of disease and for studying disease and medical care as interrelated processes." Systems theory proposes that all parts of an organization (i.e., a person, a health care system, a medical office, an endocrine system) are linked to each other so that changes in one part affect changes in the other (von Bertalanffy, 1952, 1968, 1969). Engel extolled health care providers to view their clinical work through the lens of a general systems theory.

Appendix C

Terms Commonly Used in Referring to Mental Health Professionals

Below are definitions of both adjectives and nouns that are commonly paired, in a variety of ways, to refer to mental health professionals working in a medical setting. For example, one may hear the terms *behavioral health clinician, behavioral health provider, behavioral health professional,* or other variations of a noun modified by the same adjective. Each of these terms carries a slightly different meaning depending on the context in which one is working and the meaning of the different adjectives and nouns.

Common Adjectives

Behavioral health: Suggests a broad focus on behavior and behavioral factors in health, certainly including mental disorders and conditions. This newer term may have been developed to avoid the stigma of the term *mental health* and to imply a broader scope of psychological activity related to general health care, not just mental health care. This term invites behavioral focus on such things as smoking cessation, health behaviors, and lifestyle, as well as diagnosed medical and mental health conditions.

Behavioral medicine: Often associated with a more specific focus on health care or medical conditions and physiology in medical settings, especially specialty and hospital settings. Many people associate *behavioral medicine* with a broad set of behavioral or mind-body techniques and professional study. In actual practice, this term also encompasses a focus on mental disorders, conditions, and contributing factors to a broad range of health care conditions, including mental health. Although the term *behavioral* may have originated or gained steam from the development of *behavior therapy*, there appears to be no implication now that behavioral health or behavioral medicine clinicians have to be *behaviorists* or practice *behavior therapy*, or any particular school of therapy for that matter.

Mental health: Suggests a focus on mental disorders and conditions, the various contributing factors to those conditions, and the therapies tailored to those conditions and factors. This is the more traditional term associated with mental health clinics, conditions, and practices. Although *mental health* is often distinguished from "chemical health," "chemical dependency," or "addiction," many people will use *mental health* as a blanket term for all, as we do in this book.

Common Nouns

Clinician: A clinical practitioner, assumed to be a member of a clinical profession or discipline. This term is also very general, grouping physicians, therapists, nurses, and others who see patients under one term.

Consultant: A clinician, usually a specialist, who helps primary care providers with an aspect of a case or gives expert advice or opinion on a case. When used loosely, *consultant* may refer to anyone a clinician talks to about his or her cases. In our context, the behavioral health clinician might be referred to as a *consultant* when conferring with medical physicians.

Counselor: A general term that does not require the person to be a member of a profession or considered a clinician. Generally, *counselor* is used for people who may or may not have clinical credentials but function in a helping relationship of one kind or another. The term *counselor* has a much more specific meaning in the context of the British primary care system (Hemmings, 2000).

Practitioner: A synonymous term for *clinician*.

Professional: A qualified, credentialed member of a profession. In the case of mental health *professional*, the term refers to one of a number of disciplines including psychiatry, psychology, nursing, social work, and chemical health. This very general term requires only that the person be a member in good standing of a recognized profession. This book refers to specific disciplines only when speaking to something pertaining to that discipline. Otherwise, the more general terms are used.

Provider: An alternate term for *clinician*. This term originates in the language of the "operational world" of care systems (see Chapter 3). It has become a common synonym for *clinician* but is often disliked by clinicians, probably because it is part of operational rather than clinical language. Different care systems may have different criteria for which disciplines or roles are considered providers, but all mental health professionals are generally considered providers.

Psychologist: A professional who is licensed to practice the profession of psychology. When modified by the term *health*, it refers to a professional who specializes in a broader scope of psychological activity related to general health care, not just mental health care.

Psychotherapist: A mental health professional (but usually not a psychiatrist). The term has a more specific meaning as well: a practitioner of psychotherapy. In this sense, *psychotherapist* suggests a specialization in techniques of psychotherapy, rather than general health care or behavioral health in the broader sense described earlier.

Therapist: A very general term that without any modifier can include psychotherapists, physical therapists, occupational therapists, respiratory therapists, and others. When preceded by the modifier *mental health* or *behavioral health*, the term refers to one who conducts psychotherapy. When preceded by the modifier *medical*, the term refers to one who conducts psychotherapy in a medical setting. In this book the noun *therapist* without a modifier will be used to refer to a mental health therapist.

Appendix D

Recognized Medical Specialties

Allergy and immunology: Since allergy is an immune reaction, allergists have a combined specialty title. More recently, their specialty organization has expanded its name to the American Academy of Allergy, Asthma, and Immunology, to increase their role in treating the chronic disease asthma, which is partially allergic and immunological.

Anesthesiology: Along with the traditional role of putting patients "to sleep" during surgery, anesthesiologists are now doing more regional "awake" anesthesia, for example, in obstetrics with epidural blocks. Their expertise in the area of unconscious patients has led to a greater role and a subspecialty in "critical care" in surgical intensive care units. Another subspecialty pathway for anesthesiologists has been in chronic pain management, although their focus is biological and procedural in relieving pain, often ignoring the complex psychopathology of most chronic pain patients.

Colon and rectal surgery: These surgeons limit their practice to problems of the lower bowel (cancer and other tumors), rectum, and anus (e.g., hemorrhoids).

Dermatology: Representing a branch from internal medicine, dermatologists focus only on the skin, which they proudly call the largest organ of the body. Traditionally focused on diagnosis and treatment with topical agents, many of these specialists have developed surgical and other technological expertise (e.g., laser therapy).

Emergency medicine: These physicians focus on the immediate treatment of serious problems such as trauma, heart attacks, and strokes. They cover emergency rooms 24 hours a day, 7 days a week, and like to be in radio communication with paramedical personnel in "the field." The bulk of patients who come to emergency departments have common minor problems and may be lacking a regular primary care physician, or simply want the convenience of after hours treatment.

Family practice: Family practice is the specialty developed from general practices and focuses on the care of patients of all ages in the context of the family and community. Subspecialties: Geriatric medicine, focusing on the care of the elderly, and sports medicine, focusing on problems and wellness of athletes. Family practice is considering a formal subspecialty in adolescent medicine.

Internal medicine: Internal medicine is a primary care specialty focusing on the care of adults, with an emphasis on medical rather than surgical problems. Major subspecialties:

Cardiology: These physicians focus on problems of the heart and to some degree the circulatory system. These specialists have been informally subdivided into interventional cardiologists, who perform invasive procedures such as cardiac catheterizations and angioplasty, and noninterventional cardiologists, who limit their practice to diagnosis and treatment with medication.

Endocrinology: These physicians focus on the endocrine (hormone) system and like all internists, value precise diagnosis, which guides the treatment. While the range of endocrine problems is great and complex, the most common disorders are diabetes and thyroid problems. These specialists compete to some degree with general internists and family physicians for treatment.

Gastroenterology: These physicians focus on problems of the stomach and intestines. The development of endoscopy, which is the insertion of flexible tubes to visualize the stomach and colon, has made this specialty more procedural and lucrative. However, this subspecialty is now oversupplied by practitioners in many geographical areas, and the amount of reimbursement for endoscopy has decreased.

Geriatric medicine: Geriatric specialists focus on the elderly. Internal medicine shares this subspecialty with family practice, a great example of interspecialty cooperation. With the aging of the population, geriatrics is considered in greater demand, although where the boundary of care between these subspecialists and primary care physicians should be is controversial.

Hematology/oncology: Most of these physicians focus on the medical treatment of cancers. A major change is occurring in cancer treatment such that it is moving away from use of toxic drugs that may harm the patient while treating the cancer and toward newer therapies that may enhance the patient's health and ability to fight the cancer.

Infectious disease: These physicians focus on the wide range of complex infections, especially those that occur in vulnerable populations. The treatment of AIDS has been a pervasive force in this subspecialty.

Nephrology: These physicians focus on the medical problems of the kidney and urinary tract. The care of patients on renal dialysis has been a pervasive area for nephrologists.

Pulmonary disease: These physicians focus on the problems of the lungs. Cigarette smoking and occupational exposures cause most chronic lung disease. If these causes were better controlled, these subspecialists would have less to do. They compete with primary care physicians and allergists for the treatment of asthma.

Rheumatology: These physicians focus on a loosely tied group of autoimmune problems affecting the joints and connective tissues (muscles, tendons, ligaments). The name of the subspecialty comes from *rheumatism,* an outdated term. The most common problems diagnosed by rheumatologists are rheumatoid arthritis, polymyalgia rheumatica, and systemic lupus erythematosus (lupus). The main treatments for these problems are anti-inflammatory agents, which are becoming more complex, effective, and less toxic as the biochemistry of the immune response is better understood.

Medical genetics: This small specialty is likely to explode in the 21st century with the development of extensive genetic testing and genetic therapy.

Neurological surgery: This surgical specialty may have the longest duration of training (generally nine years after medical school) and focuses on surgery of the brain and spinal column. More recently, neurological surgeons overlap with orthopedic surgeons in surgery of the vertebral bones of the neck and back.

Nuclear medicine: An imaging specialty, which grew out of radiology and uses radioactive isotopes to provide scans of organs and body parts. This specialty is declining due to newer imaging techniques such as MRI (magnetic resonance imaging) and CT (computerized tomography) scans.

Obstetrics/gynecology: One of the oldest specialties, obstetrics/gynecology focuses on the reproductive system of women. Cancers of the ovaries, uterus, and cervix are increasingly treated by gynecological oncologists. In the past, most obstetrician/gynecologists were men with a surgical orientation. Now, most in training are women, and many are interested in the broader issues of women's health care. General obstetrician/gynecologists are integrating with primary care.

Ophthalmology: This is one of the oldest specialties (described in antiquity). Ophthalmologists are increasingly surgical, leaving the care of common visual problems to optometrists, who they now frequently employ.

Orthopedic surgery: For these musculoskeletal physicians, care and surgery have become so technologically advanced that many are subspecializing in certain joints, such as the shoulder, hip, and knee. Common orthopedic problems such as sprains, strains, tendonitis, and simple fractures usually are treated by primary care physicians, who generally get along well with the "orthopods." When neck and back problems require surgery, orthopedic surgeons compete with neurosurgeons, who claim that they have greater skills and encounter fewer complications.

Otolaryngology: This specialty has had many names as it seeks to expand its territory of responsibility in the head and neck. Traditionally, otolaryngologists diagnose and treat problems of the ears, nose, and throat (ENT). The specialty has become highly advanced surgically, and most are now well-trained head-and-neck surgeons, showing their greatest skill with cancers in these areas.

Pathology: These physicians evaluate tissue and other body substances, and provide diagnostic information to treating physicians. Traditionally, pathologists perform autopsies. Now, the entire clinical laboratory is their domain, as is an expanded range of tissues (e.g., obtained by biopsies, Pap smear) and many other body substances.

Pediatrics: A primary care specialty focusing on the care of children.

Physical medicine and rehabilitation: These physicians focus on the disabled, generally those with chronic conditions such as stroke and spinal cord injuries. They are trained to assess a disabled person's needs and develop a treatment plan using a variety of providers such as physical therapists, occupational therapists, and speech pathologists.

Plastic surgery: These surgeons have two very different areas of activity: rehabilitative procedures, such as surgery after trauma or cancer surgery, and cosmetic procedures. The latter are extensively advertised and provided on a cash basis.

Preventive medicine: These physicians are trained to work in public health, focusing on populations rather than the treatment of individual patients. Physicians who train only in this specialty earn a graduate degree in public health and assume administrative positions in health care organizations, especially public health departments. They address population issues such as epidemics, environmental health, and access to care. Physicians who want to be trained for population-based roles and have clinical skills to treat patients generally obtain primary care training and then a degree in public health, with an option of dual specialization in preventive medicine.

Psychiatry and neurology: It is most interesting, especially to mental health professionals, that these two specialties have a history of a combined board certification. Although it is true that physicians specializing in one of these must have some training in the other for board certification, unfortunately this combination is in name only, as psychiatrists and neurologists have been far apart in training and practice in recent decades. Psychiatry has largely abandoned psychoanalysis and much of psychotherapy, with its major focus in research and practice now being on the biology of mental illness and pharmacotherapy. Neurologists focus specifically on the function of the brain, spinal cord, and nervous system. This mind and body split of psychiatry and neurology may be resolved with these two specialties overlapping more. Hopefully, where such overlap is relevant, such as for problems like Alzheimer's disease, the approach will be a biopsychosocial model.

Radiology: This is the imaging specialty, and the only one defined by a certain technology. Radiologists are specialists dealing with x-rays, other forms of radiation, and various imaging techniques, such as computerized tomography (CT) and magnetic resonance imaging (MRI), used for diagnosis and treatment.

Surgery: Once comprehensive specialists who were responsible for most of the body, general surgeons now work primarily in the abdomen. Some acquire additional expertise as vascular surgeons, repairing blocked blood vessels, such as in the neck and groin.

Thoracic surgery: Thoracic surgeons operate in the chest. Because of the commonness and lucrative nature of coronary bypass surgery, most of these physicians are trained for cardiothoracic surgery.

Urology: These surgeons operate on the kidney, urinary tract, and male genitalia (prostate and scrotum, including testicles). Since the prostate is the organ most commonly requiring surgery and office visits, most of their patients are men. They compete with obstetrician/gynecologists for surgery on women with incontinence problems.

Recognized Specialties in Medicine and Date of First Incorporation in the United States

Allergy & Immunology (1971)
Anesthesiology (1938)
Colon & Rectal Surgery (1935)
Dermatology (1932)
Emergency Medicine (1976)
Family Practice (1969)
Internal Medicine (1936)
Medical Genetics (1980)
Neurological Surgery (1940)
Nuclear Medicine (1971)
Obstetrics & Gynecology (1930)
Ophthalmology (1917)

Orthopedic Surgery (1934)
Otolaryngology (1924)
Pathology (1936)
Pediatrics (1933)
Physical Medicine & Rehabilitation (1947)
Plastic Surgery (1937)
Preventive Medicine (1948)
Psychiatry & Neurology (1934)
Radiology (1934)
Surgery (1937)
Thoracic Surgery (1950)
Urology (1935)

Recognized Subspecialties in Medicine, with Sponsoring Specialty and Date of First Recognition in the United States

Addiction Psychiatry (Psychiatry & Neurology, 1991)
Adolescent Medicine (Internal Medicine, 1992)
Adolescent Medicine (Pediatrics, 1991)
Blood Banking/Transfusion Medicine, (Pathology, 1972)
Cardiovascular Disease (Internal Medicine, 1937)
Chemical Pathology (Pathology, 1951)
Child and Adolescent Psychiatry (Psychiatry & Neurology, 1959)
Clinical & Laboratory Dermatological Immunology (Dermatology, 1983)
Clinical & Laboratory Immunology (Internal Medicine, 1983)
Clinical & Laboratory Immunology (Pediatrics, 1983)
Clinical Cardiac Electrophysiology (Internal Medicine, 1989)
Clinical Laboratory Immunology (Allergy & Immunology, 1983)
Clinical Neurophysiology (Psychiatry & Neurology, 1990)

Critical Care (Anesthesiology, 1985)
Critical Care Medicine (Internal Medicine, 1985)
Critical Care Medicine (Obstetrics & Gynecology, 1985)
Cytopathology (Pathology, 1988)
Dermatopathology (Dermatology, 1973)
Dermatopathology (Pathology, 1973)
Endocrinology Diabetes & Metabolism (Internal Medicine, 1971)
Forensic Pathology (Pathology, 1959)
Forensic Psychiatry (Psychiatry & Neurology, 1992)
Gastroenterology (Internal Medicine, 1938)
General Vascular Surgery (Surgery, 1982)
Geriatric Medicine (Family Practice, 1985)
Geriatric Medicine (Internal Medicine, 1985)
Geriatric Psychiatry (Psychiatry & Neurology, 1989)
Gynecologic Oncology (Obstetrics & Gynecology, 1972)

continued

Hand Surgery (Orthopedic Surgery, 1986)
Hand Surgery (Plastic Surgery, 1986)
Hematology (Internal Medicine, 1971)
Hematology (Pathology, 1955)
Immunology (Pathology, 1983)
Infectious Disease (Internal Medicine, 1971)
Interventional Cardiology (Internal Medicine, 1996)
Maternal & Fetal Medicine (Obstetrics & Gynecology, 1973)
Medical Microbiology (Pathology, 1950)
Medical Oncology (Internal Medicine, 1972)
Medical Toxicology (Emergency Medicine, 1992)
Medical Toxicology (Pediatrics, 1992)
Medical Toxicology (Preventive Medicine, 1992)
Neonatal-Perinatal Medicine (Pediatrics, 1974)
Nephrology (Internal Medicine, 1971)
Neuropathology (Pathology, 1948)
Neuroradiology (Radiology, 1994)
Nuclear Radiology (Radiology, 1972)
Otology/Neurology (Otolaryngology, 1992)
Pain Management (Anesthesiology, 1991)
Pediatric Cardiology (Pediatrics, 1961)
Pediatric Critical Care Medicine (Pediatrics, 1985)
Pediatric Emergency Medicine (Emergency Medicine, 1991)
Pediatric Emergency Medicine (Pediatrics, 1991)
Pediatric Endocrinology (Pediatrics, 1976)

Pediatric Gastroenterology (Pediatrics, 1988)
Pediatric Hematology-Oncology (Pediatrics, 1973)
Pediatric Infectious Disease (Pediatrics, 1991)
Pediatric Nephrology (Pediatrics, 1973)
Pediatric Otolaryngology (Otolaryngology, 1992)
Pediatric Pathology (Pathology, 1989)
Pediatric Pulmonology (Pediatrics, 1984)
Pediatric Radiology (Radiology, 1983)
Pediatric Rheumatology (Pediatrics, 1990)
Pediatric Surgery (Surgery, 1973)
Plastic Surgery within the Head and Neck (Otolaryngology, 1998)
Pulmonary Disease (Internal Medicine, 1937)
Reproductive Endocrinology (Obstetrics & Gynecology, 1973)
Rheumatology (Internal Medicine, 1971)
Spinal Cord Injury Medicine (Physical Medicine &Rehabilitation, 1995)
Sports Medicine (Emergency Medicine, 1991)
Sports Medicine (Family Practice, 1989)
Sports Medicine (Internal Medicine, 1992)
Sports Medicine (Pediatrics, 1990)
Surgery of the Hand (Surgery, 1986)
Surgical Critical Care (Surgery, 1985)
Undersea Medicine (Preventive Medicine, 1989)
Vascular & Interventional Radiology (Radiology, 1994)

Source: American Board of Medical Specialties, 1998. *Annual Report and Reference Handbook.* Reprinted with permission.

Appendix E

Case Rounds*:
A Group Feedback and Coaching
Practice for Clinicians

Behavioral health professionals need feedback and coaching while they are working in a medical setting. Most of this can be done in a group format where the integrated mental health professionals come together to develop their particular skills and face professionals of their own kind with issues of quality, good practice, and personal balance in roles at medical clinics. We have found the following "case rounds" format useful for this purpose, and by far the most important thing therapists do when they get together as a group.

Discussion of challenging cases brings out the accumulated knowledge and wisdom of the group. Not only do integrated mental health therapists have the opportunity and obligation to put difficult cases on the table, but they also learn from other challenging cases. Feedback and coaching is an ongoing responsibility for all clinicians and clinician leaders. As stated by one major care system: "Leave no clinician or care team alone and unaided with case problems, fears, uncertainties, or communication habits that will eventually rob them of satisfaction or affect patient care, patient relationships or staff relationships" (HealthPartners, 1993).

Case rounds is not only about the care of the patient but also about the therapist's relationship to the work and the care system. Case rounds can be the primary ongoing training modality for integrated behavioral health professionals.

---

*Based on a format used at HealthPartners Medical Group and Clinics since 1987.

All clinicians from the various mental health disciplines are combined, as one professional community. Everyone participates; thus, no one graduates from case rounds.

Case rounds start with a check-in: "Here are the cases on my mind." Criteria for putting a case on the table include when *you* have "symptoms" about the case, not just when the *patient* presents with a challenging picture. For example, a therapist should bring a case to rounds when:

1. Your hands run cold before and during the encounters.
2. You see the name on your schedule and want to go home.
3. You are relieved whenever the patient cancels an appointment.
4. You want to bury return phone calls and paperwork at the bottom of your pile, while thinking: "I'll do this when I have time to think."
5. You half-knowingly engage in behaviors likely to get you "fired" by the patient.
6. You are awash in letters from lawyers or agencies and are not sure how to respond.
7. You find it easier to refill a pain or time-off prescription than engage the patient in the larger issues involved, but you know you have to.
8. The chart is getting thicker while the patient is not improving, or you lose sleep over the case.
9. The situation brings out tensions between team members or clinic staff.
10. You would like to tell someone about a success or well-handled situation.

This list demonstrates that case rounds is clinician-centered and health care relationship–centered rather than a disease-centered consultation. In other words, case rounds is not reserved for rare clinical syndromes that comfortably challenge clinical acumen. Alternatively, case rounds is designed to help clinicians not only with their complex cases, but with ordinary clinical stress, practice patterns, blind spots, or habits that can affect patient care and service.

The goal of case rounds is for those with a case that puzzles them or gives them "cold hands" to be able to leave the room with options of what step to take next. The other, equally important, function of case rounds is to build common culture and best practices among the group. For example, therapists in case rounds captured the wisdom that experience had taught them in the form of the care management mottos that we have quoted earlier in this book (see Chapter 5, Box 5.1). These mottos express basic intellectual capital and practical wisdom of the group built up over years of practice. We find that ongoing, seriously conducted case rounds can form the cornerstone for evolving best practice, patient and clinician safety, as well as common culture across disciplines.

Case rounds is a work format, a standardized recipe for getting work done in a group. The content of the work varies, but the format for working on the content remains the same. When people learn a work format, they know what to do when they get together. There is little or no time spent trying to figure out how to get things done or what the rules and roles are for the meeting. The facilitator is responsible for preserving the work format so the group maintains a working discipline. Without this, the group reverts to mere discussion and little work gets done. The work format for case rounds has five distinct steps.

1. *Gather.* Allow a five-minute grace period after the designated starting time. This extra time allows everyone to gather, prevents rushing, preoccupation, apology, disruption, or ambivalence ("Since I'm going to be late, maybe I shouldn't go at all"). Realistic scheduling is essential. Remember that clinicians are often notorious for showing up late for meetings.

2. *Check-in.* Go around the room, giving each person a couple of minutes to say how things are going and to put a case on the agenda. Each should state how important it is to discuss the case today and how much time will be needed for it. The facilitator (sometimes one person, sometimes the responsibility rotates) will keep track, and after the check-in is complete, will negotiate time allocation. A sense of how to best spend the time quickly emerges, and the facilitator keeps the group on schedule unless the plan is specifically changed.

3. *Case presentation.* The designated first person puts a case or issue on the table, having organized his or her thoughts beforehand and providing enough information for the others: What are the relevant facts, history, signs and symptoms for why am I putting this case on the table? Are there "red flags" in this situation? What have I already tried? In what way do I need help from the group today?

4. *Resolution and moving on.* The facilitator (and hopefully the presenter and everyone else) keeps an eye on the time and gently wraps up as the time limit approaches. Not every problem is resolved, but next steps, suggestions, or new ways of thinking are presented for use. Sometimes the facilitator will ask, "Did you get enough of what you needed today to go forward?" A follow-up report or discussion of the issue at a later meeting may also be encouraged. The topics and presenters continue to cycle through in this way until time runs out.

5. *Parting.* Case rounds usually ends with a couple minutes for chitchat or consultations between individuals regarding issues that never reached the threshold for inclusion in the agenda.

In addition to the overall purpose of case rounds, there are several additional reasons why they are valuable to clinicians. For example, they help to

1. *Develop constructive approaches to managing challenging cases and to facilitate a meeting that assists with difficult cases.* Any case is welcome, but high priority is given to complex, hard-to-manage cases that challenge clinician-patient communication and health care relationship skills, especially "difficult" patient-clinician relationships. Case rounds teach clinicians how to help each other with casework that brings about challenge, complexity, frustration, uncertainty, anxiety, or avoidance. It is also a place to declare "jobs well done," which helps boost morale. It is a place to get consultation on working relationships and to address "red flag" situations before significant damage or anguish occurs.

2. *Engender a sense of community and collegiality as clinicians.* Break down the usual isolation from one another, so that clinicians can help each other maintain balance with cases that might activate personal reactions, tension, anxiety, or uncertainty about how to move forward. Clinicians "let down their hair" in an atmosphere of helpful acceptance so they don't have to hide their reactions or vulnerabilities or suffer through situations that might magnify them.

3. *Heighten awareness of the repeating themes that run through clinical work.* Case rounds gives people greater appreciation of what faces everyone, what is "normal" experience, and what works well or not in clinic practice. In a strong but informal sense, norms for clinician behavior are often created and maintained in these groups. Accumulated experience, values, and practical wisdom shapes and reinforces good health care relationship skills and care planning methods.

4. *Identify things that must be addressed outside case rounds.* Not every problem or challenge is amenable to case rounds. For example, organizational or systems barriers, personnel issues, and formal peer review typically require other approaches.

Glossary

Alternative medicine: nontraditional medical treatments including acupuncture, massage therapy, herbal medicines, and diets.

BATHE technique: a 15-minute psychosocial interview developed for physicians to screen for mental disorders.

Behavioral approach: an approach to mental health treatment that posits that behavior is maintained by the consequences to that behavior. Thus, behavior is best changed by altering consequences. This approach is characterized by the methodical and directive approach of the clinician. Classical conditioning, operant conditioning, social learning theory, and exchange theory are all under the behavioral approach umbrella. Biofeedback, parent effectiveness training, systematic desensitization, and in vivo desensitization are all common examples of mental health interventions that are based on behavioral principles. Noted scientists/therapists espousing this approach include Ivan Pavlov, B. F. Skinner, Gerald Patterson, and Richard Stuart.

Biopsychosocial: integrating biological, psychological, and social components of individuals.

Capitation: a third party payment system in which a predetermined amount of money is given to the provider for each patient assigned to the physician. The physician receives this amount of money regardless of how frequently the patient is seen, the illness that is being treated, or the type of treatment provided. The rationale to support a capitated system is that some patients will consume more than the average resources while other patients will consume less than the average. Capitated systems generally emphasize preventative medicine.

Cognitive approach: an approach to mental health treatment that emphasizes the role that thinking plays in the development and resolution of problem behaviors and interactions. If what people tell themselves about the world is not consistent with observable fact then cognition becomes distorted and problems develop. Treatment primarily involves teaching people different cognitions and self-statements. Noted theorists/therapists espousing this approach include Aaron Beck.

Comorbidity: the existence of multiple physical and/or mental illnesses within the same individual.

Confidentiality: both an ethical and legal concept that involves a restriction on the volunteering of information shared between client and therapist with certain limited exceptions including threat to self or others, child abuse, and adult elder abuse.

Cost-offset: to make something, in this case, medical care, eventually cost less by providing mental health care. Although it might initially look like it will increase costs, because it reduces overall health care costs, it saves money in the long run.

Credentialing: a process where the medical or behavioral health provider becomes authorized by a managed care company to provide services. The mental health specialist is credentialed through the primary care clinic, along with the other physicians, as a provider of the medical clinic. This works best when the managed care company does not have any local or regionally convenient behavioral health providers that could provide the care on a carve out basis.

Curb-side consultations: a colloquial term unique to collaborative health care environments. The term refers to brief, unscheduled consultations about patients or clinical issues that typically occur in the hallway as clinicians pass each other as they are moving from one appointment to the next.

DSM-IV-TR: the *Diagnostic and Statistical Manual,* 4th edition, text revision, provides a classification of psychological disorders including specific criteria that is used by clinicians to determine diagnoses of patients.

DSM-IV Primary Care Version: a shortened version of the *DSM-IV* designed for primary care physicians.

Diagnosis: process of determining whether a presenting problem meets the established criteria as determined by the *DSM-IV* for a particular psychological disorder.

Differential diagnosis: process of discriminating between possible diagnoses to determine the correct diagnosis of a patient.

Efficacy-effectiveness gap: this gap refers to the difference between laboratory created treatments with tight controls and the "real world" practice of primary care physicians.

Evidence-based medicine: an approach to medical decision making that is grounded in empirical literature. This approach emphasizes the science of medicine over the art of medicine. Physicians practicing evidence-based medicine use treatments and make treatment decisions based on the available research evidence to support the effectiveness and efficacy of the treatment.

Formulary: a list of approved prescription medications as determined by a managed care organization.

Fragmented care: the separation of patient care based on different systems to address physical and mental conditions.

Golden rule: the practice of putting the needs of patients first in the delivery of patient care.

Guild: an organization of persons with related interests, goals, etc., especially one formed for mutual aid or protection.

Humanistic approach: an approach to mental health treatment that emphasizes the human potential to achieve self-actualization. The importance of a person's unique internal (emotional) experience of the world is emphasized. Noted theorists/therapists espousing this approach include Abraham Maslow, Carl Rogers, Virginia Satir, and Carl Whitaker.

Integrated care: collaborative patient care addressing physical and mental symptoms of a patient, as well as a coordinated treatment plan between primary care physicians and mental health professionals.

Managed health care: sector of health insurance in which health care providers are administered by firms that manage the allocation of health care benefits and therefore exercise more control of health care costs.

Maneuverability: a psychotherapeutic term that refers to the clinician's ability to make treatment decisions and to maintain control over the course and direction of treatment.

Medical co-payment: the amount a patient is required to pay based on insurance benefits for a medical visit with a physician, mental health professional, and/or a prescription benefit.

Medical therapist: a trained, licensed professional providing psychotherapy and/or counseling in a medical setting. This would include the following professionals: psychiatrist, psychologist, social worker, and marriage and family therapist.

Mind-body dualism: separation between mental and physical aspects of human beings.

Neurasthenia: a pattern of symptoms including chronic fatigue, sleep disturbances, and persistent aches often linked with depression.

Primary care: integrated, accessible health care services at the point of entry, primarily in office settings that address the whole individual.

PRIME-MD: an efficient assessment instrument developed for physicians to screen for mental disorders.

Psychosocial: of or pertaining to the interaction between social and psychological factors.

Psychotropic medications: antianxiety/hypnotic drugs, antidepressants, antipsychotics, and stimulants.

Quandranary care: super specialized services such as organ transplantation.

Rounds: the process of visiting patients in the hospital to assess their progress and to reevaluate the appropriateness of treatment. These sequential visits to patients typically occur daily and with members of the treatment team. With treatment team members present, treatments can be coordinated and collaboration can be facilitated.

SDDS-PC: an efficient assessment instrument developed for physicians to screen for mental disorders.

Secondary care: health care services provided by specialists and community hospitals.

Somatization disorder: extreme and long-lasting focus on multiple physical symptoms for which no medical cause can be identified.

Subthreshold diagnoses: category of symptoms that may be overlooked in determining a patient's diagnosis, such as adjustment disorders, stress-related disorders, and NOS (not otherwise specified).

Symptoms: the presenting problem or complaints of a patient.

Tertiary care: health care services provided by subspecialists in specialized hospitals or academic health centers.

References

Alcoholics Anonymous. (1976). *Alcoholics Anonymous* (3rd ed.). New York: Alcoholics Anonymous World Services, Inc.

Allen, B., Jr., Pederson, L. L., & Leonard, E. H. (1998). Effectiveness of physicians-in-training counseling for smoking cessation in African Americans. *Journal of the National Medical Association, 90,* 597–604.

Allison, T. B., Williams, D. E., Miller, T. D., Patten, C. A., Bailey, K. R., Squires R. W., & Gau, G. T. (1995). Medical and economic costs of psychologic distress in patients with coronary artery disease. *Mayo Clinic Proceedings, 70,* 734–742.

Alpert, J. J., & Charney, E. (1973). The education of physicians for primary care. *PHS, DHEW Publication (HRA), 74,* p. 3113.

American Academy of Family Physicians (1994). *American Academy of Family Physicians official definitions related to primary care* (Report No. 302). Kansas City, MO: Author.

American Academy of Family Physicians (1998). *Facts about family practice.* Kansas City, MO: Author.

American Board of Medical Specialties. (1998). *ABMS annual report and reference handbook.* Evanston, IL: Author.

American Psychiatric Association. (2000). *Diagnostic and statistical manual of mental disorders* (4th ed., Text Revision). Washington, DC: Author.

Ancoli-Israel, S. (1996). *All I want is a good night's sleep.* St. Louis, MO: Mosby.

Anderson, C. M., & Stewart, S. (1983). *Mastering resistance: A practical guide to family therapy.* New York: Guilford.

Barrett, J. E., Barrett, J. A., Oxman, T. E., & Gerber, P. D. (1988). The prevalence of psychiatric disorders in a primary care practice. *Archives of General Psychiatry, 45*, 1100–1106.

Barsky, A. J. (1988). *Worried sick: Our troubled quest for wellness.* Boston: Little, Brown.

Baxter, L., Schwartz, J., Bergman, K., Szuba, M., Guze, B., Mazziotta, J., Alazraki, A., Selin, C., Ferng, H., Munford, P., & Phelps, M. (1992). Caudate glucose metabolic rate changes with both drug and behavior therapy for obsessive-compulsive disorder. *Archives of General Psychiatry, 49*, 681–689.

Beck, A. T. (1990). *Beck anxiety inventory.* San Antonio, TX: Psychological Corporation.

Beeder, A. B., & Millman, R. B. (1995). Treatment strategies for comorbid disorders: Psychopathology and substance abuse. In A. M. Washton (Ed.), *Psychotherapy and substance abuse: A practitioner's handbook* (pp. 76–102). New York: Guilford.

Bernard, M. E., & Rasmussen, N. H. (1999, March). *Predicting the presence of a psychiatric disorder in primary care patients.* Slide presentation at the 19th annual Society of Teachers of Family Medicine conference, Kiawah Island, South Carolina.

Beutler, L. E., Machado, P. P .P., & Neufeldt, S. A. (1994). Therapist variables. In A. E. Bergin & S. L. Garfield (Eds.), *Handbook of psychotherapy and behavior change* (4th ed.) (pp. 229–269). New York: John Wiley.

Blazer, D. G. (1993). *Depression in late life.* St. Louis: Mosby.

Blount, A. (Ed.). (1998). *Integrated primary care: The future of medical and mental health collaboration.* New York: W. W. Norton.

Bootzin, R. R., & Perlis, M. L. (1992). Nonpharmacologic treatments of insomnia. *Journal of Clinical Psychiatry, 53*, 37–41.

Boyle, R. G., O'Connor, P. J., Pronk, N. P., & Tan, A. (1998). Stages of change for physical activity, diet, and smoking among HMO members with chronic conditions. *American Journal of Health Promotion, 12*, 170–175.

Bray, J. H., & Rogers, J. C. (1997). The linkages project: Training behavioral health professionals for collaborative practice with primary care physicians. *Families, Systems, and Health, 15*, 55–63.

Broadhead, W. E., Leon, A. C., Weissman, M. M., Hoven, C. W., Barrett, J. E., Blacklow, R. S., Sheehan, D. V., & Olfson, M. (1995). Development and validation of the SDDS-PC screen for multiple mental disorders in primary care. *Archives of Family Medicine, 4*, 211–219.

Burns, B. J. (1994). Historical considerations of mental disorders in primary care. In J. Miranda, A. A. Hohmann, C. C. Attkisson, & D. B. Larson (Eds.), *Mental disorders in primary care* (pp. 16–33). San Francisco: Jossey-Bass.

Caine, E. D., Lyness, J. M., King, D. A., & Connors, L. (1994). Clinical and etiological heterogeneity of mood disorders in elderly patients. In L. S. Schneider, C. F. Reynolds, B. D. Lebowitz, & A. J. Friedhoff (Eds.), *Diagnosis and treatment of depression in late life: Results of the NIH Consensus Development Conference* (pp. 21–54). Washington, DC: American Psychiatric Press.

Campbell, T. L. (1996). Clinical trials of collaborative healthcare. *Families, Systems, and Health, 14,* 137–144.

Carney, R. M., Rich, M. W., Freedland, K. E., Saini, J., TeVelde, A., Simeone, C., & Clarke, K. (1988). Major depressive disorder predicts cardiac events in patients with coronary artery disease. *Psychosomatic Medicine, 50,* 627–633.

Carole, J., Hymel, K. P., Ritzen, A., Reinert, S. E., & Hay, T. C. (1999). Analysis of missed cases of abusive head trauma. *Journal of the American Medical Association, 281,* 621–626.

Centers for Disease Control. (1994, May 20). Cigarette smoking among adults—United States, 1992: Changes in the definition of current cigarette smoking. *Morbidity and Mortality Weekly Report* [On-line], *43*(19), 342–346. Available: http://www.cdc.gov/mmwr/preview/mmwrhtml/00033250.htm

Centers for Disease Control. (1997, December 26). Cigarette smoking among adults—United States, 1995. *Morbidity and Mortality Weekly Report* [On-line], *46*(51), 1217–1220. Available: http://www.cdc.gov/mmwr/preview/mmwrhtml/0005025.htm

Chudy, J. H. A., & Dea, R. A. (1996, March). *Integrating behavioral healthcare and primary care.* Paper presented at the Primary Care Behavioral Healthcare Summit, San Diego, CA.

Clancy, C. M., & Kamerow, D. B. (1996). Evidence-based medicine meets cost-effectiveness analysis. *Journal of the American Medical Association, 276,* 329–333.

Cohen, S., Doyle, W. J., Skoner, D. P., Rabin, B. S., & Gwaltney, J. M. (1997). Social ties and susceptibility to the common cold. *Journal of the American Medical Association, 277,* 1940–1944.

Cole-Kelly, K. (1999, March). *Healing communities: Joining together in a changing world.* Paper presented at the 19th annual Society of Teachers of Family Medicine conference, Kiawah Island, South Carolina.

Colwill, J. M. (1992). Where have all the primary care applicants gone? *New England Journal of Medicine, 326,* 387–392.

Cooper-Patrick, L. (1994). Identifying suicidal ideation in general medical patients. *Journal of the American Medical Association, 272*, 1757–1762

Coyne, J., Schwenk, T., & Fechner-Bates, S. (1995). Nondetection of depression by primary care physicians reconsidered. *General Hospital Psychiatry, 17*, 3–12.

Cummings, N. A. (1997). Behavioral health in primary care: Dollars and sense. In N. A. Cummings, J. L. Cummings, & J. N. Johnson (Eds.), *Behavioral health in primary care: A guide for clinical integration* (pp. 3–22). Madison, CT: Psychosocial Press.

Cummings, N. A., Cummings, J. L., & Johnson, J. N. (Eds.). (1997). *Behavioral health in primary care: A guide for clinical integration*. Madison, CT: Psychosocial Press.

Davis, T. F., & Heinrich, R. L. (1994). *HealthPartners clinic survey*. Unpublished data.

deGruy, F. V., III (1997). Mental health care in the primary care setting: A paradigm problem. *Families, Systems, and Health, 15*, 3–26.

deGruy, F., Columbia, L., & Dickinson, P. (1987). Somatization disorder in a family practice. *Journal of Family Practice, 25*, 45–51.

Depression Guideline Panel. (1993). *Clinical practice guideline number 5: Depression in primary care, 2: Treatment of major depression*. Rockville, MD: US Department of Health and Human Services, Agency for Health and Policy Research (93–0550).

Devesa, S. S., & Diamond, E. L. (1983). Socioeconomic and racial differences in lung cancer incidence. *American Journal of Epidemiology, 118*, 818–831.

Dietrich, A., & Eisenberg, L. (1999). Better management of depression in primary care. *Journal of Family Practice, 48*, 945–990.

Dimsdale, J. E. (1997). Symptoms of anxiety and depression as precursors to hypertention. *Journal of the American Medical Association, 277*, 574–575.

Doherty, W. J. & Baird, M. A. (1983). Family therapy and family medicine. New York: Guilford.

Doherty, W. J., & Baird, M. A. (1986). Levels of physician involvement with families. *Family Medicine, 18*, 153–156.

Doherty, W. J., & Baird, M.A. (1986). Developmental levels in family-centered medical care. *Family Medicine, 18*, 153–156.

Doherty, W. J., & Baird, M. A. (Eds.). (1987). *Family centered medical care: a clinical casebook*. New York: Guilford.

Doherty, W. J., McDaniel, S. H., & Baird, M. A. (1996). Five levels of primary care/behavioral healthcare collaboration. *Behavioral Healthcare Tomorrow, 5*, 25–27.

Doherty, W. J., & Simmons, D. S. (1996). Clinical practice patterns of marriage and family therapists: A national survey of therapists and their clients. *Journal of Marital and Family Therapy, 22*, 9–25.

Dunman, R. S., Heninger, G. R., & Nestler, E. J. (1997). A molecular and cellular theory of depression. *Archives of General Psychiatry, 54*, 597–606.

Durant, W. (1935). *The story of civilization: Vol. 1. Our Oriental heritage.* New York: Simon & Schuster.

Durant, W. (1939). *The story of civilization, Vol. 2. The life of Greece.* New York: Simon & Schuster.

Durant, W. (1944). *The story of civilization, Vol. 3. Caesar and Christ.* New York: Simon & Schuster.

Durant, W. (1956). *The story of civilization, Vol. 6. The Reformation.* New York: Simon & Schuster.

Durant, W., & Durant, A. (1963). *The story of civilization, Vol. 8. The age of Louis XIV.* New York: Simon & Schuster.

Edwards, T. M., Patterson, J., Grauf-Grounds, C., & Groban, S. (2001). Psychiatry, MFT, & family medicine collaboration: The Sharp behavioral health clinic. *Families, Systems, and Health, 19*, 25–36.

Eisenberg, D. M., Davis, R. B., Ettner, S. L., Appel, S., Wilkey, S., Van Rompay, M., & Kessler, R. C. (1998). Trends in alternative medicine use in the United States, 1990–1997. *Journal of the American Medical Association, 280*, 1569–1575.

Engel, G. L. (1977). The need for a new medical model: A challenge to biomedicine. *Science, 196*, 129–136.

Engel, G. L. (1980). The clinical application of the biopsychosocial model. *American Journal of Psychiatry, 137*, 535–544.

Engel, G. L. (1992a). The need for a new medical model: A challenge for biomedicine. *Family Systems Medicine, 10*, 317–331.

Engel, G. L. (1992b). How much longer must medicine's science be bound by a seventeenth century world view? *Family Systems Medicine, 10*, 333–346.

Ewing, J. A. (1984). Detecting alcoholism. The CAGE questionnaire. *Journal of the American Medical Association, 252*, 1905–1907.

Fawzy, F. I., Fawzy, N. W., Hyun, C. D., Elashoff, R., Guthrie, D., Fahey, J. L., & Morton, D. L. (1993). Malignant melanoma. Effects of an early structured psychiatric intervention, coping, and affective state on recurrence and survival 6 years later. *Archives of General Psychiatry, 50*, 681–689.

Feldhaus, K. M., Koziol-McLain, J., Amsbury, H. L., Norton, I. M., Lowenstein, S. R., & Abbott J. T. (1997). Accuracy of 3 brief screening questions for detecting partner violence in the emergency department. *Journal of the American Medical Association, 277,* 1357–1361.

Finkelstein, S. N., & Berndt, E. R. (1996, January). *Economics of depression: A summary and review.* Prepared for the consensus conference on the undertreatment of depression, sponsored by the National Depressive and Manic-Depressive Association, Chicago, IL.

Fischer, L. R., Heinrich, R. L., Davis, T. F., Peek, C. J., & Lucas, S. F. (1998). Mental health and primary care in an HMO. *Families, Systems, and Health, 15,* 379–391.

Fisher, L., & Ransom, D. C. (1997). Developing a strategy for managing behavioral health care within the context of primary care. *Archives of Family Medicine, 6,* 324–333.

Fitzgerald, M. A., Jones, P. E., Lazar, B., McHugh, M., & Wang, C. (1995). The midlevel provider: Colleague or competitor? *Patient Care, 29,* 20–37.

Fleming, M. F., Barry, K. L., Manwell, L. B., Johnson, K., & London, R. (1997). *Journal of the American Medical Association, 277,* 1039–1045.

Fontanarosa, P. B., & Lundberg, G. D. (1998). Editorial: Alternative medicine meets science. *Journal of the American Medical Association, 280,* 1618–1619.

Ford, E. D. (1994). Recognition and underrecognition of mental disorders in primary care. In J. Miranda, A. A. Hohmann, C. C. Attkisson, & D. B. Larson (Eds.), *Mental disorders in primary care* (pp. 186–205). San Francisco: Jossey-Bass.

Frances, R. J., & Miller, S. I. (Eds.). (1991). *Clinical textbook of addictive disorders.* New York: Guilford.

Franks, P., & Fiscella, K. (1998). Primary care physicians and specialists as personal physicians: Health care expenditures and mortality experience. *Journal of Family Practice, 47,* 105–109.

Frasure-Smith, N., Lesperance, F., & Talajic, M. (1993). Depression following myocardial infarction: Impact on 6-month survival. *Journal of the American Medical Association, 270,* 1819–1825.

Friedli, K., King, M. B., Lloyd, M., & Horder, J. (1997, December). Randomised controlled assessment of non-directive psychotherapy versus routine general-practitioner care. *The Lancet, 350,* 1662–1665.

Galuska, D. A., Will, J. C., Serdula, M. K., & Ford, E. S. (1999). Are health care professionals advising obese patients to lose weight? *Journal of the American Medical Association, 282,* 1576–1578.

Garfield, S. L. (1994). Research on client variables in psychotherapy. In A. E. Bergin & S. L. Garfield (Eds.), *Handbook of psychotherapy and behavior change* (4th ed., pp. 190–228). New York: John Wiley.

Gauthier, J. G. Bridging the gap between biological and psychological perspectives in the treatment of anxiety disorders. *Canadian Psychology/ Psychologie Canadienne, 40*, 1.

Gedenk, M., & Nepps, P. (1996). Obsessive-compulsive disorder: diagnosis and treatment in the primary care setting. *Journal of American Board of Family Practice, 10*, 349–356.

Geyman, J. P., & Hart, L. G. (1994). Primary care at a crossroads: Progress, problems and future projections. *Journal of the American Board of Family Practice, 7*, 60–70.

Gitlin, M. J. (1990). *The psychotherapist's guide to psychopharmacology.* New York: Free Press.

Glass, R. M. (1999). Treating depression as a recurrent or chronic disease. *Journal of the American Medical Association, 281*, 83–84.

Glasser, R., Rabin, B., Chesney, M., Cohen, S., & Natelson, B. (1999). Stress-induced immunomodulation: Implications for infectious diseases? *Journal of the American Medical Association, 281*, 2268–2270.

Glassman, A. H., & Shapiro, P. A. (1998). Depression and the course of coronary artery disease. *American Journal of Psychiatry, 155*, 4–11.

Goetzel, R. Z., Anderson, D. R., Whitmer, R. W., Ozminkowski, R. J., Dunn, R. L, Wasserman, J., & Health Enhancement Research Organization (HERO) Research Committee (1998). The relationship between modifiable health risks and health care expenditures: An analysis of the multi-employer HERO health risk and cost database. *Journal of Occupational and Environmental Medicine, 40*, 1–12.

Goldstein, E., Lobel, J., Faigeles, B., & DeCarlo, P. (1998). Sources of information for HIV prevention program managers: A national survey. *AIDS Education and Prevention, 10*, 63–74.

Gonzalez, S., Steinglass, P., & Reiss, D. (1989). Putting illness in its place: Discussion groups for families with chronic medical illness. *Family Process, 28*(1), 69–87.

Goode, E. (1998, November 24). How much therapy is enough? It depends. *The New York Times*, Section F, p. 1.

Goodwin, F. J., & Jamison, K . R. (1990). *Manic-depressive illness.* New York: Oxford University Press.

Griffith, J. L., & Griffith, M. E. (1994). *The body speaks: Therapeutic dialogues for mind-body problems.* New York: Basic.

Grunebaum, M. (1996). Predictors of missed appointments for psychiatric consultations in a primary care clinic. *Psychiatric Services, 47,* 848–852.

Gullette, E. C. D., Blumenthal, J. A., Babyak, M., Jiang, W., Waugh, R. A., Frid, D. J., O'Connor, C. M., Morris, J. J., & Krantz, D. S. (1997). Effects of mental stress on myocardial ischemia during daily life. *Journal of the American Medical Association, 277,* 1512–1526.

Guyatt, G. H. (1993). Editorial: Users' guides to the medical literature. *Journal of the American Medical Association, 270,* 2096–2097.

Guyatt, G., & Rennie, D. (2002). *Users' guide to the medical literature: A manual for evidence-based clinical practice.* Chicago: AMA Press.

Haber, J. D., & Mitchell, G. E. (Eds.). (1998). *Primary care meets mental health: Tools for the 21st century.* Providence, RI: Behavioral Health Resource Press.

Halvorson, G. (1993). *Strong medicine.* New York: Random House.

Hamberger, L. K., Ambuel, B., Marbella, A., & Donze, J. (1998). Physician interaction with battered women: The women's perspective. *Archives of Family Medicine, 7,* 575–582.

Hamilton, M. (1959). The assessment of anxiety states. *British Journal of Medical Psychology, 32,* 50–55.

Handley, M. R., & Stuart, M. E. (1994). An evidence-based approach to evaluating and improving clinical practice: Guideline development. *HMO Practice, 8,* 10–19.

HealthPartners. (1993). *Core practice of medical managers* [internal training material]. Minneapolis, MN: Author.

Hellman, C. J., Budd, M., Borysenko, J., McClelland, D. C., & Benson, H. (1990). A study of the effectivness of two group behavioral medicine interventions for patients with psychosomatic complaints. *Behavioral Medicine, 16,* 165–173.

Hemmings, A. (2000). A systematic review of the effectiveness of brief psychological therapies in primary health care. *Families, Systems, and Health, 18,* 279–313.

Hirschfield, R. M. A., & Russell, J. M. (1997). Assessment and treatment of suicidal patients. *The New England Journal of Medicine, 337*(16), 910–916.

Hirschfield, R., Keller, M., Panice, S., Arons, B., Barlow, D., Davidoff, F., Endicott, J., Froom, J., Goldstein, M., Gorman, J., Guthrie, D., Marek, R., Mayrer, T., Meyer, R., Phillips, K., Ross, J., Schwenk, T., Sharfstein, S., Thase, M., & Wyatt, R. (1997). The National Depressive and Manic-Depressive Association consensus statement on the undertreatment of depression. *Journal of the American Medical Association, 277,* 333–340.

Hoddes, E., Zarcone, V., Smythe, H., Phillips, R., & Dement, W. C. (1973). Quantification of sleepiness: A new approach. *Psychophysiology, 10*, 431–436.

Holmes, T. H., & Rahe, R. H. (1968). The social readjustment rating scale. *Journal of Psychosomatic Research, 11*, 213–218.

House, J. S., Landis, K. R., & Umberson, D. (1988). Social relationships and health. *Science, 241*, 540–545.

Howard, K. I., Kopta, S. M., Krause, M. S., & Orlinsky, D. E. (1986). The dose effect relationship in psychotherapy. *American Psychologist, 41*, 159–164.

Hurt, R. D., Dale, L. C., Fredrickson, P. A., Caldwell, C. C., Lee, G. A., Offord, K. P., Lauger, G. G., Marusic, Z., Neese, L. W., & Lundberg, T. G. (1994). Nicotine patch therapy for smoking cessation combined with physician advice follow-up. One-year outcome and percentage of nicotine replacement. *Journal of the American Medical Association, 271*, 595–600.

Hymowitz, N., Sexton, M., Ockene, J., & Grandits, G. (1991). Baseline factors associated with smoking cessation and relapse. MRFIT research. *Preventive Medicine, 20*, 590–601.

Institute of Medicine. (1978). *A manpower policy for primary health care.* Washington, DC: National Academy Press.

Institute of Medicine. (1996). *Primary care: America's health in a new era.* Washington, DC: National Academy Press.

Isham, G. (1997, November/December). Population health and HMOs: The Partners for Better Health experience. *HealthCare Forum Journal*, 36–39.

Jackson, S. W. (1999). *Care of the psyche: A history of psychological healing.* New Haven, CT: Yale University Press.

Jenny, C., Hymel, K. P., Ritzen, A., Reinert, S., & Hag, T. (1999). Analysis of missed cases of abusive head trauma. *Journal of the American Medical Association, 281*, 621–626.

Jonas, B. S., Franks, P., & Ingram, D. D. (1997). Are symptoms of anxiety and depression risk factors for hypertension? *Archives of Family Medicine, 6*, 43–49.

Kaplan, R. (2000, March). The reservoir of illness. Presentation at Society of Teachers of Family Medicine conference, San Diego, CA.

Kashner, T. M., Rost, K., & Cohen, B. (1995). Enhancing the health of somatization disorder patients: Effectiveness of short-term group therapy. *Psychosomatics, 36*, 462–470.

Kassirer, J. P. (1994). Access to specialty care. *New England Journal of Medicine, 331*, 115–152.

Katon, W., Von Korff, M., Lin, E., Walker E., Simon, G. E., Bush, T., Robinson, P., & Russo, J. (1995). Collaborative management to achieve treatment guidelines. *Journal of the American Medical Association, 273*, 1026–1031.

Katon, W., Lin, E., Von Korff, M., Bush, T., Walker, E., Simon, G., & Robinson, P. (1994). The predictors of persistence of depression in primary care. *Journal of Affective Disorders, 31,* 81–90.

Katon, W., Robinson, P., Von Korff, M., Lin, E., Bush, T., Ludman, E., Simon, G., & Walker, E. A. (1996). Multifaceted intervention to improve treatment of depression in primary care. *Archives of General Psychiatry, 53,* 924–932.

Katon, W., Von Korff, M., Lin, E., Bush, T., Lipscomb, P. & Russo, J. (1992). A randomized trial of psychiatric consultation with distressed high utilizers. *General Hospital Psychiatry, 14,* 86–98.

Katzelnick, D. (1997, May). Integrated care and cost offset services for depressed and somaticizing high utilizers. In *Institute for Behavioral Healthcare conference: How to design and implement your primary care behavioral health integration program* (pp. 81–148). San Francisco: Institute for Behavioral Healthcare.

Keller, M. B., Klerman, G. L., Lavori, P. W., Fawcett, J. A., Corywll, W., & Endicott, J. (1982). Treatment received by depressed patients. *Journal of the American Medical Association, 248,* 1848–1855.

Keller, M. B., Lavori, P. W., Klerman, G. L., Andreason, N. C., Endicott, J., Coryell, W., Fawcett, J., Rice, J. P., & Hirschfeld, R. M. (1986). Low levels and lack of predictors of somatotherapy and psychotherapy received by depressed patients. *Archives of General Psychiatry, 43,* 458–466.

Keller, V. F., & Carroll, J. G. (1994). *A new model for physician-patient communication.* West Haven, CT: Miles Institute for Health Care Communication.

Kempe, C. H., Silverman, F. N., Steele, B. F., Droegemueller, W., & Silver, H. K. (1962). The battered child syndrome. *Journal of the American Medical Association, 181,* 17–24.

Kessler, R. C., McGonagle, K. A., Zhao, S., Nelson, C. B., Hughes, M., Eshleman, S., Wittchen, H., & Kendler, K. S. (1994). Lifetime and 12-month prevalence of *DSM-III-R* psychiatric disorders in the United States: Results from the national comorbidity survey. *Archives of General Psychiatry, 51,* 8–19.

Kiecolt-Glaser, J. K., & Glaser, R. (1995). Psychoneuroimmunology and health consequences: Data and shared mechanisms. *Psychosomatic Medicine, 57,* 269–274.

Kimmel, P. L., Peterson, R. A., Weins, K. L., Simmens, S. J., Boyle, D. H., Cruz, I., Umana, W. O., Allgre, S., & Veis, J. H. (1995). Aspects of quality of life in hemodialysis patients. *Journal of the American Society of Nephrology, 6,* 1418–1426.

Kitchens, J. M. (1994). Does this patient have an alcohol problem? *Journal of the American Medical Association, 272,* 1782–1787.

Kleinman, A. (1988). *The illness narratives: Suffering, healing and the human condition*. New York: Basic.

Klinkman, M. S., & Okkes, I. (1998). Mental health problems in primary care: A research agenda. *Journal of Family Practice, 47*, 379–384.

Kocsis J. H., Friedman, R. A., Markowitz, J. C., Leon, A. C., Miller, N. L., Gniwesch, L., & Parides, M. (1996). Maintenance therapy for chronic depression: A controlled clinical trial of desipramine. *Archives of General Psychiatry, 53*, 769–774.

Kroenke, K., & Mangelsdorff, D. (1989). Common symptoms in ambulatory care: Incidence, evaluation, therapy and outcome. *American Journal of Medicine, 86*, 262–266.

Krupnick, J. L., Sotsky, S. M., Simmens, S., Moyer, J., Elkin, I., Watkins, J., & Pilkonis, P. A. (1996). The role of the therapeutic alliance in psychotherapy and pharmacotherapy outcome: Findings in the National Institute of Mental Health treatment of depression collaborative research program. *Journal of Consulting and Clinical Psychology, 64*, 532–539.

Law, M., & Tang, J. L. (1995). An analysis of the effectiveness of interventions intended to help people stop smoking. *Archives of Internal Medicine, 155*, 1933–1941.

Lazarus, R. S. (1985). The trivialization of distress. In J. C. Rosen & L. J. Solomon (Eds.), *Preventing health risk behaviors and promoting coping with illness: Vol. 8 of the Vermont Conference on the Primary Prevention of Psychotherapy* (pp. 279–298). Hanover, NH: University Press of England.

Leon, A. C., Olfson, M., Broadhead, W. E., Barrett, J. E., Blacklow, R. S., Keller, M. B., Higgins, E. S., & Weissman, M. M. (1995). Prevalence of mental disorders in primary care. *Archives of Family Medicine, 4*, 857–861.

Leplege, A., & Hunt, S. (1997). The problem of quality of life in medicine. *Journal of the American Medical Association, 278*, 47–50.

Levenson, J. L. (1992). Psychosocial interventions in chronic medical illness: An overview of outcome research. *General Hospital Psychiatry, 14S*, 43S–49S.

Leventhal, J. M. (1999). The challenges of recognizing child abuse: Seeing is believing. *Journal of the American Medical Association, 281*, 657–659.

Levinson, W., Roter, D. L., Mullooly, J. P., Dull, V. T., & Frankel, R. M. (1997). Physician-patient communication: The relationship with malpractice claims among primary care physicians and surgeons. *Journal of the American Medical Association, 277*, 553–559.

Liftik, J. (1995). Assessment. In S. Brown (Ed.), *Treating alcholism* (pp. 57–94). San Francisco: Jossey-Bass.

Linden, W., Stossel, C., & Maurice, J. (1996). Psychosocial interventions for patients with coronary artery disease: A meta-analysis. *Archives of Internal Medicine, 156,* 745–752.

Lipchik, G. L. (1998). Anxiety or mood disorders often accompany chronic tension headache. *Modern Medicine, 66,* 20.

Lipowski, Z. J. (1988). Somatization: The concept and its clinical application. *American Journal of Psychiatry, 145,* 1358–1368.

Little, D. N., Hammond, C., Kollisch, D., Stern, B., Gagne, R., & Dietrich, A. J. (1998). Referrals for depression by primary care physicians. *Journal of Family Practice, 47,* 375–377.

Lucas, S. F., & Peek, C. J. (1997). A primary care physician's experience with integrated behavioral health care: What difference has it made? In N. A. Cummings, J. L. Cummings, & J. N. Johnson (Eds.), *Behavioral health in primary care: A guide for clinical integration* (pp. 371–398). Madison, CT: Psychosocial Press.

Lynch, J. W., Kaplan, G. A., & Shema, S. J. (1997). Cumulative impact of sustained economic hardship on physical, cognitive, psychological, and social functioning. *New England Journal of Medicine, 337,* 1889–1895.

Maorin, C. M. (1993). *Insomnia: Psychological assessment and management.* New York: Guilford.

Maruish, M. (Ed.). (2000). *Handbook of psychological assessment in primary care settings.* Mahwaeh, NJ: Lawrence Erlbaum.

Mauksch, L. B., Tucker, S. M., Katon, W. J., Russo, J., Cameron, J., Walker, E., & Spitzer, R. (2000). Mental illness, functional impairment, and patient preferences for collaborative care in an uninsured, primary care population. *Journal of Family Practice, 50,* 41–47.

Maxmen, J. S., & Ward, N. G. (1995). *Essential psychopathology and its treatment* (2nd ed.). New York: W.W. Norton.

May, R. R. (1987). Therapy in our day. In J. K. Zeig (Ed.), *The evolution of psychotherapy* (pp. 212–219). New York: Brunner/Mazel.

Mayfield, D., McLeod, G., & Hall, P. (1974). The CAGE questionnaire: Validation of a new alcoholism screening instrument. *American Journal of Psychiatry, 131,* 1121–1123.

McCauley, J., Kern, D. E., Kolodner, K., Dill, L., Schroeder, A. F., DeChant, H. K., Ryden, J., Derogatis, L. R., & Bass, E. B. (1997). Clinical characteristics of women with a history of childhood abuse: Unhealed wounds. *Journal of the American Medical Association, 277,* 1362–1368.

McCulloch, J., Ramesar, S., & Peterson, H. (1998). Psychotherapy in primary care: The BATHE Technique. *American Family Physician, 57,* 2131–2134

McDaniel, S., Campbell, T., & Seaburn, D. (1990) *Family-oriented primary care: A manual for medical providers*. New York: Springer-Verlag.

McDaniel, S., Campbell, T., & Seaburn, D. (1995). Principles for collaboration between health and mental health providers in primary care. *Family Systems Medicine, 13*, 283–298.

McDaniel, S. H., Hepworth, J., & Doherty, W. J. (1992). *Medical family therapy: A biopsychosocial approach to families with health problems*. New York: Basic.

McDaniel, S., Hepworth, J., & Doherty, W. (1997). *The shared experience of illness*. New York: Basic.

McEwen, B. S. (1998). Protective and damaging effects of stress mediators. *New England Journal of Medicine, 338*, 171–179.

Miller, R. H., & Luft, H. S. (1994). Managed care plan performance since 1980. *Journal of the American Medical Association, 271*, 1512–1519.

Miller, R. H., & Luft, H. S. (1997). Does managed care lead to better or worse quality of care? *Health Affairs, 16*, 7–25.

Miller, W. R., & Rollnick, S. (1991). *Motivational interviewing: Preparing people to change addictive behavior*. New York: Guilford.

Miranda, J., Hohmann, A. A., Attkisson, C. C., & Larson, D. B. (Eds.). (1994). *Mental disorders in primary care*. San Francisco: Jossey-Bass.

Mokdad, A. H., Serdula, M. K., Dietz, W. H., Bowman, B. A., Marks, J. S., & Koplan, J. P. (1999). The spread of the obesity epidemic in the United States, 1991–1998. *Journal of the American Medical Association, 282*, 1519–1522.

Moran, M. (1999). Psychosocial disorders in primary care: A hidden problem. *American Medical News, 42*, 43–44.

Morin, C. M., Colecchi, C., Stone, J., Sood, R., & Brink, D. (1999). Behavioral and pharmacological therapies for late-life insomnia: A randomized controlled trial. *Journal of the American Medical Association, 281*, 991.

Mullin, F. (1998). The "Mona Lisa" of health policy: Primary care at home and abroad. *Health Affairs, 17*(2), 118–126.

Murphy, G. P., & Sciandra, R. (1983). Helping patients withdraw from smoking. *New York State Journal of Medicine, 83*, 1353–1354.

Murray, C. L. J., & Lopez, A. D. (1997). Global mortality, disability, and the contribution of risk factors: Global burden of disease study. *Lancet, 349*, 1436–1442.

Must, A., Spadano, J., Coakley, E. H., Field, A. E., Colditz, G., & Dietz, W. H. (1999). The disease burden associated with overweight and obesity. *Journal of the American Medical Association, 262*, 1523–1529.

Mynors-Wallis, L. M., Gath, D. H., Lloyd-Thomas, A. R., & Tomlinson, D. (1995). Randomized controlled trial comparing problem solving treatment with amitriptyline and placebo for major depression in primary care. *British Medical Journal, 310*, 441–445.

Nace, E. P., & Isbell, P. G. (1991). Alcohol. In R. J. Frances & S. I. Miller (Eds.), *Clinical textbook of addictive disorders* (pp. 43–68). New York: Guilford.

Narrow, W. F., Regier, D. A., Rae, D. S., Manderscheid, R. W., & Locke, B. Z. (1993). Use of services by persons with mental and addictive disorders: Findings from the National Institute of Mental Health Epidemiologic Catchment Area Program. *Archives of General Psychiatry, 50*, 95–107.

National Committee on Quality Assurance (1998). *HEDIS health plan employer and data information set (1998 report)*. Washington, DC: Author.

National Committee on Quality Assurance (1999). *NCQA standards for managed care organizations (1998 and 1999 eds.)*. Washington, DC: Author.

National Institutes of Health Technology Assessment Panel. (1996). Integration of behavioral and relaxation approaches into the treatment of chronic pain and insomnia. *Journal of the American Medical Association, 276*, 313–318.

Ness, D. E., & Ende, J. (1994). Denial in the medical interview: Recognition and management. *Journal of the American Medical Association, 272*, 1777–1781.

Norcross, J. C. (Ed.). (1986). *Handbook of eclectic psychotherapy*. New York: Brunner/Mazel.

Norcross, J. C. (Ed.). (1987). *Casebook of eclectic psychotherapy*. New York: Brunner/Mazel.

O'Connor, P. J., & Pronk, N. P. (1998). Integrating population health concepts, clinical guidelines, and ambulatory medical systems to improve diabetes care. *Journal of Ambulatory Care Management, 21*, 170–175.

O'Connor, P. J., Rush, W. A., & Pronk, N. P. (1997). Database system to identify biological risk in managed care organizations: Implications for clinical care. *Journal of Ambulatory Care Management, 20*, 4.

O'Connor, P. J., Solberg, L. I., & Baird, M. (1998). The future of primary care: The enhanced primary care model. *Journal of Family Practice, 47*, 62–67.

Oldham, J. M. (1994). Personality disorders: current perspectives. *Journal of the American Medical Association, 272*, 1770–1776.

Olds, D., Henderson, C. R., Cole, R., Eckenrode, J., Kitzman, H., Luckey, D., Pettitt, L., Sidora, K., Morris, P., & Powers, J. (1998). Long-term effects of nurse home visitation on children's criminal and antisocial behavior: Fifteen-year follow-up of a randomized controlled trial. *Journal of the American Medical Association, 280*, 1238–1244.

Ormel, J., Koeter, M., Brink, W., & Williege, G. (1991). Recognition, management, and course of anxiety and depression in general practice. *Archives of General Psychiatry, 48*, 700–706.

Ormel, J., Von Korff, M., Bedirhan Ustun, T., Pini, S., Korten, A., & Oldehinkel, T. (1994). Common mental disorders and disability across cultures: Results from the WHO collaborative study on psychological problems in general health care. *Journal of the American Medical Association, 272*, 1741–1748.

Ornish, D., Scherwitz, L. W., Billings, J. H., Gould, K. L., Merritt, T. A., Sparler, S., Armstrong, W. T., Ports, T. A., Kirkeeide, R. L., Hogeboom, C., & Brand, R. J. (1998). Intensive lifestyle changes for reversal of coronary heart disease. *Journal of the American Medical Association, 280*, 2001–2007.

Osler, W. (1932). *Aequanimitas* (3rd ed.). Philadelphia: Blakiston.

Othmer, E., & DeSouza, C. A. (1985). A screening test for somatization disorder. *American Journal of Psychiatry, 142*, 1146–1149.

Patterson, J. (2001). Training: The missing link in creating collaborative care, *Family Systems and Health, 19*, 1–5.

Patterson, J., & Bischoff, R. (1999). [Family functioning: *DSM-IV* diagnosis and quality of life in a primary care population]. Unpublished raw data.

Patterson, J., Bischoff, R., & McIntosh-Koontz, L. (1997). Training issues in integrated care. In A. Blount (Ed.), *Integrated primary care: The future of medical and mental health collaboration* (pp. 261–283). New York: W. W. Norton.

Patterson, J., Bischoff, R., Scherger, J., & Grounds, C. (1996). University family therapy training and a family medicine residency in a managed care setting. *Family Systems and Health, 14*, 5–16.

Patterson, J., Hayworth, M., & Turner, C. (2000). The family therapists' guide to spirituality. *Journal of Marital and Family Therapy, 26*, 198–209.

Patterson, J., & Magulac, M. (1994). Pharmacology for family therapists. *Journal of Marital and Family Therapy, 20*, 151–171.

Patterson, J., McIntosh-Koontz, L., Baron, M., & Bischoff, R. (1997, October). Curriculum changes to meet challenges: Preparing MFT students for managed care settings. *Journal of Marital and Family Therapy, 23*, 445–460.

Patterson, J., & Scherger, J. (1995). A critique of health care reform in the United States: Implications for training and practice in marriage and family therapy. *Journal of Marital and Family Therapy, 21*, 127–135.

Patterson, J., Williams, L., Grounds, C., & Chamow, L. (1998). *Essential skills in family therapy*. New York: Guilford

Pear, R. (1999, June 21). Future bleak for bill to keep health records confidential. *The New York Times* [On-line]. Available: www.nytimes.com

Pear, R. (2000, January 24). U.S. Health officials reject plan to report media mistakes. *The New York Times* [On-line]. Available: www.nytimes.com

Peek, C. J. (1988, October). Status dynamics and the integration of medical and mental health care. Paper presented at the Tenth Annual Meeting of the Society for Descriptive Psychology, Boulder, CO.

Peek, C. J., & Heinrich, R. L. (1995). Building a collaborative healthcare organization: From idea to invention to innovation. *Family Systems Medicine*, *13*(3/4), 327–342.

Peek, C. J., & Heinrich, R. L. (1998). Integrating primary care and behavioral health in a healthcare organization: From pilot to mainstream. In A. Blount (Ed.), *Integrated primary care: The future of medical and mental health collaboration* (pp. 167–202). New York: W. W. Norton.

Peek, C. J., & Heinrich, R. L. (2000). Integrating behavioral health and primary care. In M. Maruish (Ed.), *Handbook of psychological assessment* (pp. 59–61). Mahwah, NJ: Lawrence Erlbaum Associates.

Pincus, H. A., Tanielian, T. L., Marcus, S. C., Olfson, M., Zarin, D. A., Thompson, J., & Zito, J. M. (1998). Prescribing trends in psychotropic medications. *Journal of the American Medical Association*, *279*, 526–531.

Pingitore, D., & Sansone, R. (1998). Using DSM-IV primary care version: A guide to psychiatric diagnosis in primary care. *American Family Physician*, *58*, 1347–1352.

Plocher, D., & Kongstvedt, P. R. (1998). *Best practices in medical management*. New York: Aspen.

Pollin, I. (1992). A model for counseling the medically ill: The Linda Pollin Foundation approach. *General Hospital Psychiatry*, *12*, 1–2.

Pollin, I. (1994). *Taking charge: Overcoming the challenge of long-term illness*. New York: Times Books.

Pollin, I. (1995). *Medical crisis counseling: Short-term therapy for long-term illness*. New York: W. W. Norton.

Prochaska, J. O., & DiClemente, C. C. (1983). Stages and processes of self-change of smoking: Toward an integrative model. *Journal of Consulting and Clinical Psychology*, *51*, 390–395.

Prochaska, J. O., & DiClemente, C. C. (1992). Stages of change in the modification of problem behaviors. *Progressive Behavior Modification*, *28*, 183–218.

Prochaska, J. O., Norcross, J. C., & DiClemente, C. C. (1994). *Changing for good*. New York: Avon.

Pronk, N., & O'Connor, P. (1997). Systems approach to population health improvement. *Journal of Ambulatory Care Management*, *20*, 24–31.

Pronk, N., O'Connor, P., Isham, G., & Hawkins, C. (1997). Building a patient registry for implementation of health promotion initiatives: Targeting high-risk individuals. *HMO Practice, 11*, 1.

Pronk, N. P., Boyle, R. B., & O'Connor, P. J. (1998). The association between physical fitness and diagnosed chronic conditions in health maintenance association members. *American Journal of Health Promotion, 12*, 300–306.

Pronk, N. P., Tan, A. W. H., & O'Connor, P. J. (1998). Obesity, fitness, willingness to communicate. *Medicine and Science in Sports and Exercise, 31*(11), 1535–1543.

Putman, A. O. (1990) Organizations. In A. O. Putman & K. E. Davis (Eds.), *Advances in descriptive psychology* (pp. 11–46). Ann Arbor, MI: Descriptive Psychology Press.

Rakel, R. E., (1993). Insomnia: Concerns of the family physician. *Journal of Family Practice, 36*, 551–558.

Ransom, D. C. (1997). Mental healthcare in the primary care setting. *Families, Systems and Health, 15*, 27–36.

Rapaport, M. H. (1999, March). *Understanding quality of life in anxiety disorders*. Paper presented at the 19th national conference of the Anxiety Disorders Association of America, San Diego, CA.

Rasmussen, N. H., & Avant, R. F. (1989). Somatization disorder in family practice. *American Family Physician, 40*, 206–214.

Rasmussen, N. H. & Agerter (1999, March) Somatization disorder: A perplexing and challenging problem. Paper presented at the Society of Teachers of Family Medicine, Kiawah Island, SC.

Reeve, C. (1999). *Still me*. New York: Ballantine.

Regier, D., Goldberg, I., & Taube, C. (1978). The de facto U.S. mental health services system. *Archives of General Psychiatry, 35*, 685–693.

Regier, D. A., Narrow, W. E., Rae, D. S., Manderscheid, R. W., Locke, B. Z., & Goodwin, F. K. (1993). The de facto U.S. mental and addictive disorders service system: Epidemiologic catchment area prospective 1-year prevalence rates of disorders and services. *Archives of General Psychiatry, 50*, 85–94.

Reust, C. E., Thomlinson, R. P., & Lattie, D. (1999). Keeping or missing the initial behavioral health appointment: A qualitative study of referrals in a primary care setting. *Families Systems and Health, 17*(4), 399–411.

Revicki, D. A., Simon, G. E., Chan, K., Keton, W., & Heiligenstein, J. (1998). Depression, health-related quality of life, and medical cost outcomes of receiving recommended levels of antidepressant treatment. *Journal of Family Practice, 47*, 446–452.

Reynolds, C. F., Frank, E., Perel, J. M., Imber, S. D., Comes, C., Miller, M. D., Mazumdar, S., Houck, P. R., Dew, M. A., Stack, J. A., Pollock, B. G., & Kupfer, D. J. (1999). Nortriptyline and interpersonal psychotherapy as maintenance therapies for recurrent major depression. *Journal of the American Medical Association, 281,* 39–45.

Richard, D. (1998). What counts as evidence? A personal odyssey into alternative care. *Archives of Family Medicine, 7,* 598–599.

Robinson, R. G., Starr, L. B., & Price, T. R. (1984). A two-year longitudinal study of post-stroke mood disorders: Prevalence and duration at six months follow-up. *British Journal of Psychiatry, 144,* 256–262.

Rodriguez, M. A., Bauer, H. M., McLoughlin, E., & Grumbach, K. (1999). Screening and intervention for intimate partner abuse: Practices and attitudes of primary care physicians. *Journal of the American Medical Association, 282*(5), 468–474.

Rolland, J. S. (1984). Toward a psychosocial typology of chronic and life-threatening illness. *Family Systems Medicine, 2,* 245–262.

Rolnick, S. J., & O'Connor, P. J. (1997). Assessing the impact of clinical guidelines: Research lessons learned. *Journal of Ambulatory Care Management, 20,* 47–55.

Rosenberg, M., Powell, K., & Hammond, R. (1997, May 28). Applying science to violence prevention. *Journal of the American Medical Association,* 1641–1642.

Rosenblatt, R. A., Hart, L. G., Baldwin, L. M., Chan, L., & Schneeweiss, R. (1998). The generalist role of specialty physicians: Is there a hidden system of primary care? *Journal of the American Medical Association, 279,* 1364–1370.

Rosenthal, E. (1997, March 16). The H.M.O. catch: When healthier isn't cheaper. *The New York Times,* pp. 1, 4.

Rosenthal, S. B. (1995). Living with low vision: A personal and professional perspective. *American Journal of Occupational Therapy, 49,* 861–864.

Rosser, W. W. (1996). Approach to diagnosis by primary care clinicians and specialists: Is there a difference? *Journal of Family Practice, 42,* 139–144.

Roter, D. L., Hall, J. A., Kern, D. E., Barker, L. R., Cole, K. A., & Roca, R. P. (1995). Improving physicians' interviewing skills and reducing patients' emotional distress. *Archives of Internal Medicine, 155,* 1877–1884.

Rumsfeld, J. S., MaWhinney, S., McCarthy, M., Jr., Shroyer, A. L. W., VillaNueva, C. B., O'Brien, M., Moritz, T. E., Henderson, W.G., Grover, F. L., Sethi, G. K., & Hammermeister, K. E. (1999, April). Health-related quality of life as a predictor of mortality following coronary artery bypass graft surgery. *Journal of the American Medical Association, 281,* 1298.

Sackett, D. L., Rosenberg, W. M. C., Gray, J. A. M., Haynes, R. B., & Richardson, W. S. (1996). Evidence based medicine: what it is and what it isn't. *British Medical Journal, 312,* 71–72.

Schulberg, H. C., Katon, W. J., Simon, G. E., & Rush, A. J. (1999). Best clinical practice: Guidelines of managing major depression in primary medical care. *Journal of Clinical Psychiatry, 60,* 19–26.

Schulberg, H. C., Katon, W., Simon, G. E., & Rush, A. J. (1998). Treating major depression in primary care practice. *Archives of General Psychiatry, 55,* 1121–1127.

Schulberg, H. C., & Pajer, K. A. (1994). Treatment of depression in primary care. In J. Miranda, A. A. Hohmann, C. C. Attkisson, & D. B. Larson (Eds.), *Mental disorders in primary care* (pp. 259–286). San Francisco: Jossey-Bass.

Schulz, M., & Masek, B. (1996). Medical crisis intervention with children and adolescents with chronic pain. *Professional Psychology: Research and Practice, 27,* 121–129.

Schurman, R. A. (1985). The hidden mental health network. *Archives of General Psychiatry, 42,* 89–94.

Schwade, S. (1999, March). Depressive symptoms may reflect normal sadness. *Family Practice News, 29,* 22.

Seaburn, D. B., Lorenz, A. D., Gunn, W. B., Gawinski, B. A., & Mauksch, L. B. (1996). *Models of collaboration: A guide for mental health professionals working with health care practitioners.* New York: Basic.

Selye, H. (1976). *The stress of life.* New York: McGraw Hill.

Selzer. M. L. (1971). The Michigan Alcoholism Screening Test: The quest for a new diagnostic instrument. *American Journal of Psychiatry, 127,* 89–94.

Sempos, C., Cooper, R., Kovar, M. G., & McMillen, M. (1988). Divergence of the recent trends in coronary mortality for the four major race-sex groups in the United States. *American Journal of Public Health, 78,* 1422–1427.

Serdula, M. L., Mokdad, A. H., Williamson, D. F., Galuska, D. A., Mendlein, J. M., & Heath, G. W. (1999) *Journal of the American Medical Association 282*(14), 1353–1358.

Shapiro, D. E., & Koocher, G. P. (1996). Goals and practical considerations in outpatient medical crises intervention. *Professional Psychology: Research and Practice, 27,* 109–120.

Shapiro, S., Skinner, E. A., Kesler, L. G., Von Korff, M., German, P. S., Tischler, G. L., Leaf, J., Benham, L., Cottler, L., & Regier, D. A. (1984). Utilization of health and mental health services: Three epidemioloigcal catchment area sites. *Archives of General Psychiatry, 41,* 971–978.

Shea, M. T., Elkin, I., Imber, S. D., Sotsky, S. M., Watkins, J. T., Collins, J. F., Pilkonis, P. A., Beckham, E., Glass, D. R., & Dolan, R. T. (1992). Course of depressive symptoms over follow-up. *Archives of General Psychiatry, 49,* 782–787.

Shi, L. (1992). The relationship between primary care and life chances. *Journal of Healthcare for the Poor and Underserved, 3,* 321–335.

Shochat, T., Umphress, J., Israel, A. G., & Ancoli-Israel, S. (1999). Insomnia in primary care patients. *Sleep, 22*(2), S359–S365.

Shortell, S. M., Gillies, R. R., & Anderson, D. A. (1994, Winter). The new world of managed care: Creating organized delivery systems. *Health Affairs, 13,* 46–64.

Simon, G., Von Korff, M., & Barlow, W. (1995). Health care costs associated with depressive and anxiety disorders in primary care. *Archives of General Psychiatry, 52,* 850–856.

Simon, G. E., Von Korff, M., Heilgenstein, J. H., Revicki, D. A., Grothaus, L., Katon, W., & Wagner, E. H. (1996). Initial antidepressant choice in primary care. *Journal of the American Medical Association, 275,* 1897–1902.

Simon, G. E., & Von Korff, M. (1997). Is the integration of behavioral health into primary care worth the effort? A review of the evidence. In N. A. Cummings, J. L. Cummings, & J. N. Johnson, (Eds.), *Behavioral health in primary care: A guide for clinical integration* (pp. 145–162). Madison, CT: Psychosocial Press.

Slavney, P. R., & Teitelbaum, M. L. (1985). Patients with medically unexplained symptoms: *DSM-III* diagnoses and demographic characteristics. *General Hospital Psychiatry, 7,* 21–25.

Smith, G. R., Jr., Monson, R. A., & Ray, D. C. (1986). Psychiatric consultation in somatization disorder. *New England Journal of Medicine, 314,* 1407–1413.

Smith, G. R., Jr., Rost, K., & Kashner, T. M. (1995). A trial of the effect of a standardized psychiatric consultation on health outcomes and costs in somatizing patients. *Archives of General Psychiatry, 52,* 238–243.

Smyth, J. M., Stone, A., Hurewitz, A., & Kaell, A. (1999). Effects of writing about stressful experiences on symptom reduction in patients with rheumatoid arthritis: A randomized trial. *Journal of the American Medical Association, 281,* 1304–1309.

Sobel, D. S. (1995). Rethinking medicine: Improving health outcomes with cost-effective psychosocial interventions. *Psychosomatic Medicine, 57,* 234–244.

Sobel, D. S. (1997, November). *Improving health outcomes through collaborative care: "Out of the box" healthcare strategies.* Paper presented at the Third National Primary Care Behavioral Healthcare Summit, Chicago, IL.

Spiegel, D. (1993). Psychosocial intervention in cancer. *Journal of the National Cancer Institute, 85,* 1198–1205.

Spiegel, D. (1999). Healing words: Emotional expression and disease outcome. *Journal of the American Medical Association, 281,* 1328–1329.

Spiegel, D., Bloom, J. R., & Kraemer, H. C. (1989). Effect of psychosocial treatment on survival of patients with metastatic breast cancer. *Lancet, 2,* 888–891.

Spiegel, J. S., Rubenstein, L. U., Scott, B., & Brook, R. H. (1983). Who is the primary physician? *New England Journal of Medicine, 308,* 1208–1212.

Spielman, A. J., Saskin, P., & Thorpy, M. J. (1987). Treatment of chronic insomnia by restriction of time in bed. *Sleep, 10,* 45–56.

Spitzer, R. L., Williams, J. B.W., Kroenke, M., Linzer, F., deGruy, F., Hahn, S., Brady, D., & Johnson, J. (1994). Utility of a new procedure for diagnosing mental disorders in primary care: The PRIME-MD 1000 study. *Journal of the American Medical Association, 272,* 1749–1756.

Stampfer, M. J., He, F. B., Manson, J.E., Rimm, E. B., & Willett, W. C. (2000, July 6). Primary prevention of coronary heart disease in women through diet and lifestyle. *The New England Journal of Medicine, 343*(1), 16–22.

Starfield, B. (1991). Primary care and health: A cross-national comparison. *Journal of the American Medical Association, 266,* 2268–2271.

Starkstein, S. E., & Robinson, R. G. (1989). Affective disorders and cerebral vascular disease. *British Journal of Psychiatry, 154,* 170–182.

Starr P. (1982). *The social transformation of American medicine.* New York: Basic.

Strosahl, K. (1997). Building primary care behavioral health systems that work: A compass and a horizon. In N. A. Cummings, J. L. Cummings, & J. N. Johnson (Eds.), *Behavioral health in primary care: A guide for clinical integration* (pp. 37–60). Madison, CT: Psychosocial Press.

Strosahl, K. (1998). Integrating behavioral health and primary care services: The primary mental health model. In A. Blount (Ed.), *Integrated primary care: The future of medical and mental health collaboration* (pp. 139–166). New York: W. W. Norton.

Stuart, S., & Noyes, R., Jr. (1999). Attachment and interpersonal communication in somatization. *Psychosomatics, 40,* 34–43.

Terry, L. L. (1983). The Surgeon General's first report on smoking and health. A challenge to the medical profession. *New York State Journal of Medicine, 83,* 1254–1255.

Unutzer, J., Patrick, D. L., Simon, G., Grembowski, D., Walker, E., Ruter, C., & Katon, W. (1997). Depressive symptoms and the cost of health services in HMO patients age 65 years and older: A 4-year prospective study. *Journal of the American Medical Association, 277,* 1618–1623.

von Bertalanffy, L. (1952). *General systems theory.* New York: John Wiley.

von Bertalanffy, L. (1968). *General system theory—Foundations, development, applications* (4th ed.). New York: George Braziller.

von Bertalanffy, L. (1969). *Organismic psychology and systems theory.* Barre, MA: Clark University Press.

Von Korff, M. (1996). *Mental illness and addiction in the general medical sector: Incidence, prevalence, utilization patterns and outcomes.* Paper presented at the Primary Care Behavioral Healthcare Summit, San Diego, CA.

Von Korff, M., Gruman, J., Schaeffer, J., Curry, W., & Wagner, E. (1997). Collaborative management of chronic illness. *Annals of Internal Medicine, 127,* 12.

Von Korff, M., Ormel, J., Katon, W., & Lin, E. H. (1992). Disability and depression among high utilizers of health care: A longitudinal analysis. *Archives of General Psychiatry, 49,* 91–100.

Wagner, E., Austin, T., & Von Korff, M. (1996). Organizing care for patients with chronic illness. *Milbank Quarterly, 74,* 4.

Wallace, B. C. (1995). Women and minorities in treatment. In A. M. Washton (Ed.), *Psychotherapy and substance abuse: A practitioner's handbook* (pp. 470–492). New York: Guilford.

Wang, J. M. (2001, February 1). Exercise as effective as medication for depression: Study of 133 patients over age 50. *Family Practice News, 31*(3), 8.

Warner, K. E. (1986). Smoking and health implications of a change in the federal cigarette excise tax. *Journal of the American Medical Association, 255,* 1028–1032.

Washton, A. M. (1995). Clinical assessment of psychoactive substance use. In A. M. Washton (Ed.), *Psychotherapy and substance abuse: A practitioner's handbook* (pp. 23–54). New York: Guilford.

Weissman, M. M., Olfson, M., Leon, A. C., Broadhead, W. E., Gilbert, T. T., Higgins, E. S., Barrett, J. E., Blacklow, R. S., Keller, M., & Hoven, C. (1995). Brief diagnostic interviews (SDDS-PC) for multiple mental disorders in primary care. *Archives of Family Medicine, 4,* 220–227.

Weissman, M., Bland, R. C., Canino, G. J., Faravelli, C., Greenwald, S., Hwu, H. G., Joyce, P. R., Karam, E. G., Lee, C. J., Lellouch, J., Lepine, J. P., Newman, S. C., Rubio-Stipec, M., Wells, J. C., Wickramaratne, P. J., Wittchen, H., & Yeh, E. K. (1996). Cross-national epidemiology of major depression and bipolar disorder, *Journal of the American Medical Association, 276,* 293–299.

Wells, K. B., Stewart, A., Hays, R. D., Burnam, M., Rogers, W., Daniels, M., Berg, S., Greenfield, S., & Ware, J. (1989). The functioning and well being of depressed patients: Results from the medical outcomes study. *Journal of the American Medical Association, 262,* 914–919.

Wetzler, H. P., & Cruess, D. F. (1985). Self-reported physical health practices and health care utilization: Findings from the Health Interview Study. *American Journal of Public Health, 75,* 1329–1330.

White, K. L. (1967). Primary medical care for families—Organization and evaluation. *New England Journal of Medicine, 277,* 847–852.

White, K. L., Williams, T. F., & Greenberg, B. G. (1961). The ecology of medical care. *New England Journal of Medicine, 265,* 885–893.

Williams, R. B., & Chesney, M. A. (1993). Psychosocial factors and prognosis in established coronary artery disease: The need for research on interventions. *Journal of the American Medical Association, 270,* 1860–1861.

Wilson, I. B., & Cleary, P. D. (1995). Linking clinical variables with health-related quality of life. A conceptual model of outcomes. *Journal of the American Medical Association, 273,* 59–65.

Wright, S. M., Kern, D. E., Kolodner, K., Howard, D., & Branccti, F. (1998). Attributes of excellent attending-physician role models. *New England Journal of Medicine, 339,* 1986–1993.

Zeig, J. K. (1987a). Introduction: The evolution of psychotherapy—fundamental issues. In J. K. Zeig (Ed.), *The evolution of psychotherapy* (pp. xv–xxvi). New York: Brunner/Mazel.

Zeig, J. K. (Ed.). (1987b). *The evolution of psychotherapy.* New York: Brunner/Mazel.

Zeig, J. K. (Ed.). (1995). *The evolution of psychotherapy revisited.* New York: Brunner/Mazel.

Zimberg, S. (1995). The elderly. In A. M. Washton (Ed.), *Psychotherapy and substance abuse: A practitioner's handbook* (pp. 413–427). New York: Guilford.

Index